M000012875

101 AMAZING USES for CINNAMON

TO MY MOM,
THE CHINESE HOME-REMEDY QUEEN,
AND TO KATE,
WITHOUT WHOM THIS BOOK
WOULDN'T BE POSSIBLE.

Copyright © 2021 by Nancy Chen
All rights reserved.

Published by Familius LLC, www.familius.com

Familius books are available at special discounts, whether for bulk purchases for sales promotions or for family or corporate use. For more information, contact Premium Sales at 559-876-2170 or email orders@familius.com.

Reproduction of this book in any manner, in whole or in part, without written permission of the publisher is prohibited.

Library of Congress Cataloging-in-Publication Data
2020946268

Print ISBN 978-1-64170-291-1
Ebook ISBN 978-1-64170-363-5

Edited by Peg Sandkam
Cover design by Carlos Guerrero
Book design by Maggie Wickes and David Miles

Printed in the United States of America

10 9 8 7 6 5 4 3 2 1
First Edition

101 AMAZING USES for CINNAMON

CINNAMON CAN BE USED AS A
MEMORY BOOSTER,
TO MAKE A COLD REMEDY,
TREAT ACNE & ECZEMA.

By
Nancy Chen

FAMILIUS

CONTENTS

INTRODUCTION

CINNAMON: THE SPICE OF THE WORLD

If there's one spice most people have in their pantry, it's cinnamon. This fragrant brown spice is found in recipes and treatments around the world, including in South-African fried cinnamon rolls, Dutch cookies, Caribbean chicken, Sudanese tea, traditional Chinese medicine, and much more.

Its history dates back to the ancient Chinese, Egyptians, and Romans—to name just a few major civilizations—where they used it as medicine, for embalming, and more. As time went on, Western powers began to see the value of cinnamon and even fought wars to gain control over the spice trade.

Today, we can get cinnamon quite easily from our local grocery stores (no fighting or traveling needed!). In this book, you'll discover the amazing uses of cinnamon. Not only will this book provide some of these feel-good, international cinnamon recipes, but you will also learn how cinnamon can be used to treat an incredible variety of health conditions, create natural beauty products, and solve common household problems.

....

WHAT IS IT?

Cinnamon comes from the inner bark of evergreen *Cinnamomum* trees in the laurel family; different trees provide the different types of cinnamon you can find in the grocery store.

There are two main types of cinnamon: cassia and Ceylon. Although both are beneficial and have that classic sweet-and-spicy flavor, they are harvested differently and have slightly different tastes and chemical compounds.

Cassia cinnamon is the more common type of cinnamon. It has a more intense flavor than Ceylon cinnamon, so you only need a little to lend flavor to your cooking or baking. Ceylon cinnamon— which many people call "true" cinnamon—is harder to find and more expensive.[1] Its delicate flavor lacks the intense spiciness that cassia cinnamon has.

All types of cinnamon get their flavor and familiar aroma from cinnamaldehyde, an organic compound found in *Cinnamomum* trees. This compound is responsible for many of cinnamon's benefits, like its antimicrobial and antifungal properties.[2] Its most concentrated form is in essential oil—essential oil made from cinnamon bark is 90 percent cinnamaldehyde.

....

WHERE DID IT COME FROM?

Cinnamon has been used throughout the ages by some of the largest civilizations in the world and was once more valuable than gold. It was so highly regarded at one point, cinnamon was considered a suitable gift for rulers! There were four main producers of cinnamon in ancient times: Sri Lanka (the source of Ceylon cinnamon), Ethiopia, India, and China. This cinnamon was then distributed around the world.

The ancient Egyptians used cinnamon to embalm their dead bodies, likely due to cinnamon's antibacterial properties. In the Bible, cinnamon was noted to have been used in anointing oil and for other religious ceremonies. Emperor Nero of ancient Rome was rumored to have burned an entire year's supply of cinnamon at his wife's funeral in 65 CE.

By the end of the fifteenth century, the Portuguese discovered Sri Lanka and established a monopoly on the cinnamon trade there, even building a fort to cement their hold. Meanwhile, Venetian traders held control of the cinnamon brought by Arab traders from Asia. As demand for cinnamon began to rise, the Dutch began looking for new ways to gain hold of and profit from the cinnamon trade like their fellow Europeans.

During the seventeenth century, the Dutch managed to seize control of the prospering cinnamon trade by allying with the island of Kandy. They maintained a tight hold, using the Dutch East India Company to export cinnamon to Europe. At the time, it was the company's most profitable spice.

By the time the British gained control from the Dutch in 1796,[3] the monopoly on cinnamon was rapidly declining. People had discovered new places to grow cinnamon, and the value plummeted.

That leads us to the present, when cinnamon is a commonly used and much enjoyed spice.

WHAT'S THE BEST WAY TO BUY AND STORE CINNAMON?

Cinnamon comes in a variety of forms: bark, powder, stick, and essential oil. Cinnamon bark is the hardest to find—it's only available at some online specialty spice retailers and small spice stores. Bark is the most "unprocessed" form of cinnamon; it is ground up to produce cinnamon powder and rolled up to form cinnamon sticks. Because bark is a little hard to use, the other forms of cinnamon are recommended.

You can find ground cinnamon and cinnamon sticks in the baking aisle of your grocery store. Like most spices, ground cinnamon and cinnamon sticks can be stored in your pantry for a relatively long period of time. Cinnamon powder maintains its freshness for about six months (after that, it loses its potency but doesn't go bad), while cinnamon sticks can be stored for longer (about two years). Both forms should be kept in a sealed glass jar and away from heat and light.

Lastly, cinnamon essential oil can be found at some grocery stores, many health stores, and online. Essential oils are distilled from a whole plant and are its most potent form. Just a drop or two can make a big difference in beauty products and household uses.

WHAT'S THE BEST WAY TO USE CINNAMON?

Ground cinnamon is ready to use as is—you can sprinkle it on your recipes, in various homemade household cleaners, and even in DIY beauty products. Careful though: A little goes a long way!

Cinnamon sticks are good if you want to mull wine—it helps lend its sweet flavor and aroma to the liquid it's sitting in. Because the sticks are not broken down like powder is, the sticks impart less potent flavor.

When using essential oils, remember that it's best to use a carrier oil due to essential oils' high potency. Cinnamon essential oils, and even cinnamon itself, can be found in a variety of lotions, fragrances, and other common cosmetic products.

You may also see cinnamon supplements—these are higher-dosage capsules containing cinnamon and other ingredients encased in a pill. They are advertised as natural health products that can help boost your immune system, support your body with powerful antioxidants, and help with brain function and memory. They can be purchased online and at health food stores. Refer to the recommended dosage on the bottle and consult your doctor if you have any questions.

HOW MUCH SHOULD I USE?

The recommended amount of cinnamon consumed or used depends on the age and size of the person. Additionally, some people are more sensitive to cinnamon than others. This is because cassia cinnamon contains high coumarin levels, which may cause liver problems in people who consume it in high dosages. The typical recommended dosage of ground cinnamon for adults is 1–4 grams each day, which equals 0.38–1.54 teaspoons. If using cinnamon essential oil, the daily dosage ranges from 0.05 to 0.22 milliliters.[4]

Babies under six months should not be given cinnamon. After the first six months, small amounts of cinnamon can be sprinkled onto their food to help with the taste.

IS TAKING/USING CINNAMON SAFE?

Cinnamon is considered to be a safe food additive. However, it is a spice that should be taken in moderation. Too much cinnamon can drop the blood sugar dangerously low, causing dizziness and fatigue. If too much is inhaled at once, cinnamon can cause breathing problems and even suffocation. Cinnamon is thought to be safe for pregnant women in small amounts, but high dosages should be avoided. As always, consult with your doctor before using.

Even when using cinnamon topically, it's best to use it in moderation. If too much cinnamon is used on your skin, it can cause burning or irritation. It's recommended you test a small amount of any product that uses cinnamon on a patch of your arm before applying it to large areas, especially the face.

There are mixed reviews from scientists and doctors on whether cinnamon capsules are recommended because there is no regulation on supplements and no knowledge of whether the amount of cinnamon in the capsules has a positive effect on your body.

CHAPTER 1

FOR THE HOME COOK IN YOU

1. UPGRADE YOUR COFFEE

If you're trying to wean yourself off sugar in your coffee, a sprinkle of cinnamon can make a huge difference. Cinnamon adds natural sweetness, helping you skip the sweeteners or lessen the amount you typically need. (This also helps you lower the number of calories in your daily cup of coffee if you're trying to lose weight.)

Beyond simply adding extra flavor to your coffee, adding cinnamon to your morning cup of joe can also help boost your health. Cinnamon has been shown to improve memory, is a rich source of antioxidants, and can help reduce cholesterol.[1] So if you have a habit of drinking coffee regularly, adding cinnamon to it can be an easy way to get these benefits.

There are a couple of ways to add cinnamon to coffee, ranging from quite simple to more elaborate. The easiest way is to just sprinkle some on top of your cup of coffee, latte, or cappuccino. Kicking things up a notch, if you're brewing your own coffee, you can easily infuse cinnamon into the brewing process: add half of the ground coffee, then some cinnamon to taste (a pinch should do it!), and top it off with the rest of the coffee. This works for pour-over, French press, or drip coffee.

If you want to get really fancy, you can create your own cinnamon syrup. It has less artificial sugar than many store-bought coffee syrups and allows you to sweeten your coffee exactly as you want—not too much and not too little.

You can also create a keto coffee with cinnamon, a dose of high-quality fat, and brewed coffee. This type of "rocketfuel" or "Bulletproof" coffee was popularized by Bulletproof founder Dave

Asprey, who was inspired by the yak-butter tea he was offered when traveling through the Himalayas.[2] It's designed to be a breakfast replacement because it's highly satiating and both nutrient- and calorie-dense. Coffee made in this style has a high concentration of fats and a low carb count, making it a staple for keto and low-carb eaters alike.

CINNAMON COFFEE SYRUP

1 cup brown sugar (packed lightly)
1 cup water
1 teaspoon cinnamon

1. Combine all ingredients in a pot.
2. Cook over medium heat, slowly whisking, until the sugar is dissolved. Turn the heat down to a simmer if the mixture starts to boil.
3. Once the sugar is dissolved, remove the pot from the heat and let the mixture cool.
4. Store in a glass jar and use in your coffee as desired.

ROCKETFUEL KETO COFFEE

1 cup hot coffee
1 teaspoon cinnamon
1 tablespoon coconut oil or MCT oil
1 tablespoon ghee or butter (can use cocoa butter or vegan butter for a dairy-free option)
1 tablespoon coconut cream
1 scoop of collagen powder (optional)

1. Combine all ingredients in a blender.
2. Blend on high until creamy.
3. Pour into a cup and enjoy!

2. MAKE SPREADS

People have been making butter for centuries. This beloved spread had a few different purposes, ranging from medicinal in Ancient Rome (used for coughs), spiritual in India (ghee was offered to the god Krishna), and as a celebratory food in the Bible (when angels were offered a feast that included butter).[3]

The process of making butter is simple—it's just churned milk. Whether it's made by using a butter churn like Laura Ingalls Wilder or by shaking a goat hide filled with milk like the Syrians, something wonderful happens when you intensely mix up milk.

These days, getting butter is easy. You can buy it at nearly any grocery store or farmer's market. It's used in a variety of ways, from baking and cooking to spreading on top of bread and melting on top of pancakes. And if you've ever been to a really fancy restaurant, you might notice the butter is different. Sometimes it's spiced or flavored with herbs; sometimes it's whipped.

Cinnamon can help spice up any regular spread, whether it's butter or nut butter, by giving it an extra cozy kick. These two recipes are amazing when enjoyed on any sweet treat, like freshly baked bread, waffles, or pancakes.

CINNAMON BUTTER

1/2 cup butter or vegan butter, room temperature (if you use salted butter, omit the pinch of salt)

1/3 cup honey

2 teaspoons cinnamon

Pinch of salt

1. Combine all ingredients in a medium bowl.
2. Whisk together until smooth. If desired, add more cinnamon and honey to taste.
3. Store in a glass jar and serve with bread, pastries, etc.

FRESHLY GROUND SNICKERDOODLE NUT BUTTER

1 cup almonds
1 cup cashews
1/2 cup macadamia nuts
Sea salt, to taste
Cinnamon, to taste
Honey, to taste (optional; omit if following a low-sugar diet)

1. Combine all nuts in a food processor or high-speed blender.
2. Process or blend until creamy. You may have to stir occasionally to prevent the mixture from sticking to the blades.
3. Slowly add the sea salt, cinnamon, and honey to taste. Continue blending until everything is completely mixed.
4. Store in an airtight jar and use as desired.

3. PRESERVE FOOD

Before the invention of modern-day refrigerators, people used a variety of methods to preserve food. This included canning, which was invented by Nicolus Appert in 1809 CE. Appert was a French scientist who stored food in glass jars that he then sterilized using heat.[4] Fast-forward to 2000 CE, when chemical preservatives were invented. But even methods as simple as using vinegar can help preserve food longer than its natural spoiling point.

As the number of chemical additives began to get larger and

NUTRITION

BEAUTY

HEALTH

HOME

larger in preserved food, people began to seek alternatives. This is where cinnamon comes in—cinnamon essential oil has been shown to help prevent bacteria and other microbes from spoiling food due to its high antimicrobial properties. Research suggests cinnamon essential oil can be used as a food preservative, or even incorporated into food packaging, to reduce bacterial contamination.[5]

If you are creating preserves at home (such as jam), you can add cinnamon to your recipe to help extend the food's shelf life.

4. MAKE COZY DRINKS

Adding cinnamon to your drinks is an easy way to incorporate more of this sweet spice and its benefits into your diet. It also helps make ordinary drinks—like homemade nut milk—taste a little more special. There are a variety of ways you can use cinnamon in your drinks:

Mexican Superfood Hot Chocolate: Hot chocolate (or "drinking chocolate") was first drunk in Mexico as early as 500 BCE.[6] In 1500 BCE, Cortez brought it from Mexico back to Spain, where they replaced the vanilla with cinnamon and added sugar, making it more similar to the hot chocolate we know and love today.[7]

Better-than-Coffeeshop Cinnamon Chai: Chai tea, or *masala chai* ("spiced tea"), has been around for thousands of years. It was created as an Indian Ayurvedic drink (more on Ayurveda later!) and actually did not contain black tea at first. After the arrival of the British—who set up tea plantations in India—black tea began to be incorporated into the *masala chai*.[8] The unique blend of fragrant spices (of which cinnamon is an important part) and tea continues to be a popular drink in coffee shops and tea houses today.

Baby's Dream Cinnamon Milk: Warm milk before bed is an age-old remedy to help people sleep. Adding cinnamon to it can help even more by relieving cramps, if you have them. And adding honey replenishes your liver with glycogen to help keep you asleep. This drink also has natural sugar, which raises your insulin levels slightly and allows the amino acid tryptophan to enter your brain, which sets off a chain reaction that helps get you to sleep. This powerhouse combination of ingredients will help you sleep just like a baby!

Homemade Cinnamon Almond Milk: Many nut milks are made with gums and fillers to help stabilize the milk and make it last longer. However, nothing compares to freshly made nut milk—it's rich, creamy, and tastes real. The addition of cinnamon gives it an extra-special flavor you just can't find in most store-bought nut milks.

MEXICAN SUPERFOOD HOT CHOCOLATE

16 ounces milk of choice (I recommend coconut or macadamia)

2 tablespoons cacao powder

2 squares 100% dark chocolate, chopped

1 teaspoon cinnamon

1 teaspoon cayenne

1 teaspoon vanilla extract

1 tablespoon honey or maple syrup

Bonus for Adults: Add 1/2 a shot of mezcal to make it a boozy, smoky hot chocolate!

1. Heat all ingredients except the vanilla extract and sweetener (and mezcal, if using) in a small pan over medium heat until it's at a boil.

2. Remove from the heat and add the vanilla extract and sweetener of choice. (If you're making it a boozy hot chocolate, add the mezcal now.)

3. Whisk thoroughly to combine, ensuring the chopped pieces of chocolate are melted.

4. Pour into a mug and enjoy.

BETTER-THAN-COFFEESHOP CINNAMON CHAI

1 whole cinnamon stick
1 whole star anise
5-7 green cardamom pods
3-4 whole cloves
5-7 whole black peppercorns
1 teaspoon ground nutmeg
1 tablespoon grated ginger
2 cups water
3 tea bags of black tea (or 3 tablespoons loose-leaf black tea)
2 cups milk of choice (I recommend cashew or macadamia)
1 tablespoon maple syrup, brown sugar, or sweetener of choice (optional)

1. Crush whole spices into smaller pieces with a mortar and pestle. If you don't have one, use a heavy object—such as a pan—over a cutting board.

2. Add the spices, ginger, and water to a pot. Heat over medium heat until it's at a boil.

3. Lower the heat and simmer for 15 minutes.

4. Add the black tea. Continue simmering for 5 minutes.

5. Add your milk of choice. Stir to mix and continue simmering for another 3 minutes.

6. Turn off the heat and allow the mixture to steep for 10 minutes.

7. If adding sweetener, add and stir to combine.

8. Strain before serving.

BABY'S DREAM CINNAMON MILK

12 ounces milk of choice

1 teaspoon cinnamon

1 tablespoon honey

1. Heat the milk in a small pot until it's almost boiling.
2. Add the cinnamon and honey. Whisk thoroughly.
3. Pour into a mug and enjoy! Best enjoyed before bed.

Note: *This is called "Baby's Dream" to help you sleep like a baby. Cinnamon is not recommended for infants under six months of age. Honey is not recommended for infants under the age of one year.*

HOMEMADE CINNAMON ALMOND MILK

1 cup almonds (raw, organic)

2 cups distilled water (plus additional water for soaking)

2 pitted dates

1 teaspoon ground cinnamon

1 teaspoon vanilla extract

Maple syrup, to taste

1. In a large bowl, cover the almonds in distilled water and soak overnight.
2. Drain and rinse the nuts.
3. Pour all the ingredients into a high-speed blender.
4. Blend on high until the milk looks rich and creamy.
5. Taste the blend—if desired, you can add more cinnamon, vanilla, and/or maple syrup.
6. Pour the blend into a nut milk bag and squeeze into a large bowl. You may have to do this multiple times, so having another set of hands around could be helpful. If you don't have a nut milk bag, cover a fine mesh strainer with a cheesecloth and pour the nut milk into the strainer to strain the pulp out.

Squeeze the cheesecloth at intervals to make sure all the milk gets out.

7. Store in a clean glass jar for up to a week and enjoy!

5. MAKE AYURVEDIC RECIPES

Ayurveda is an ancient holistic practice that originated in India over five thousand years ago. The word is Sanskrit for "the science of life," and the practice is commonly regarded as "the mother of all healing."[9]

Today, Ayurvedic principles are still practiced by the health-and-wellness community, holistic practitioners, and many other people. There are three types of energy: *vata* (associated with movement; elements space and air), *pitta* (associated with our metabolic system; elements fire and water), and *kapha* (associated with the structure of our body, like bones and muscles; elements earth and water). People can be categorized into each energy type, or *dosha*, based on their characteristics.

Ayurveda focuses on the balance of energy; once you know your energy type, you can follow a style of eating designed to keep your body balanced. Specific spices and herbs—like ginger, cinnamon, and turmeric—help to keep this balance with their warming or cooling properties. For example, cinnamon is helpful in "increasing metabolic fire." It is also described as a "hot potency," meaning it has a heating effect.[10]

Cinnamon can be used in a variety of ways, but one of the most popular Ayurvedic foods is golden milk, which you can create with golden milk paste. It's based on a traditional Ayurvedic recipe that has been used over the years to help support both your body and your mind.[11]

GOLDEN MILK PASTE

1 cup water
1/4 cup turmeric powder
1 tablespoon cinnamon powder
1 teaspoon fresh ginger, grated
1 teaspoon black pepper
1 teaspoon cardamom or nutmeg (optional)
3 tablespoons coconut oil

1. Combine all ingredients except the coconut oil in a small pot.
2. Simmer until the ingredients thicken and start to form a paste.
3. Remove from the heat and allow to cool for 5 minutes.
4. Stir in the coconut oil until it's completely integrated into the paste.
5. Pour into a clean jar and store in the refrigerator for up to three weeks. You can use this to make golden milk (add a tablespoon of the paste to 16 ounces of dairy-free milk), add to curry or dessert, or even mix a small amount into your dog's food to give him or her the same benefits as it'll give you.

6. UPGRADE YOUR COCKTAILS

The word *cocktail* was first coined by a British newspaper in 1798, but it wasn't truly known until 1806, when *The Balance and Columbian Repository* of New York defined it as "a stimulating liquor composed of any kind of sugar, water and bitters, vulgarly called a bittered sling."[12]

Today, cocktails are prevalent at bars, restaurants, and even home dinner parties. They range from basic to singularly interesting. While it can seem intimidating to watch a bartender make a cocktail (they move so fast!), these drinks are actually quite easy to make at home.

The easiest way to incorporate cinnamon in your cocktails is to stir it with a cinnamon stick—this pairs best with any cocktail that has a little cinnamon already in it or a whiskey-based cocktail. If you want to try your hand at a more complicated drink, adding cinnamon to more unique cocktails helps add an extra layer of taste; it works especially well with wintery drinks and in mulled wine.

WELCOMING WINTER SANGRIA

1 bottle of Cabernet Sauvignon or other dry red wine
1/4 cup Grand Marnier
1/4 cup brandy
1/4 cup cranberry juice
1/2 cup frozen cranberries
1/4 cup pomegranate seeds
2 tablespoons agave or honey
1 orange, halved and then sliced
1 lime, sliced
1 pear, sliced
1 Granny Smith apple, sliced
2 cinnamon sticks, plus more for garnish
1 cup seltzer water
Rosemary, to garnish

1. Combine all ingredients except for the seltzer water and rosemary in a large pitcher.

2. Stir thoroughly.
3. Cover and place in the refrigerator for at least 2 hours.
4. Add the seltzer water right before serving.
5. Pour over ice or serve chilled. Add rosemary sprigs and extra cinnamon sticks for garnish.

PITCHER PINEAPPLE MARGARITAS WITH CINNAMON-SUGAR RIM

FOR MARGARITA:
2 cups pineapple juice
1 cup tequila
1 cup Triple Sec, or any other orange liqueur
1/2 cup lime juice

FOR RIM:
2 tablespoons fine sugar
1 teaspoon cinnamon
1/2 teaspoon nutmeg
Pinch of salt
1 lime, sliced

FOR GARNISH:
Fresh pineapple
Cinnamon sticks

1. Combine all margarita ingredients together in a large pitcher and stir thoroughly.
2. On a small plate, combine the sugar, cinnamon, nutmeg, and salt.
3. Rub the rims of four glasses with lime. Dip the rims of the glasses in the cinnamon sugar and thoroughly coat.
4. Pour the margarita into the cups over ice, garnish with pineapple and cinnamon sticks if desired, and enjoy.

NUTRITION

BEAUTY

HEALTH

HOME

APPLE CINNAMON MULLED WINE

1 bottle of dry red wine

1 cup apple cider

1/4 cup brandy

4 tablespoons honey or maple syrup (or sweetener of choice), to taste

1 orange, sliced, plus extra for garnish

8 whole cloves

5 thin slices fresh ginger

2 cinnamon sticks, plus extra for garnish

2 whole star anise, plus extra for garnish

1. Add all ingredients, except the cinnamon sticks and star anise, to a large pot and stir.

2. Cook on medium heat until the mulled wine begins to simmer.

3. Reduce the heat to low and cover. Allow the wine to simmer for 30 minutes to an hour.

4. Use a mesh strainer to strain the wine into a large bowl.

5. If desired, add in extra sweetener.

6. Serve in mugs and garnish with cinnamon sticks, sliced orange rounds, and star anise.

7. CREATE A SPECIAL SPICE MIX

Spices have been used since the hunter-gatherer era—primarily for preserving food and their medicinal properties.[13] They quickly became more valuable—they were traded as early as the thirteenth century and were as sought after as gold.[14] In fact, powerful European countries hired explorers to sail across the ocean to countries like India in search of establishing spice trade routes.

This began the struggle of Western world powers trying to gain a piece of the coveted spice trade in the East and kick-started globalization.[15]

These days, spices are fairly easy to find—you can pick them up from any grocery store. However, special spice blends are a little less common. These blends have been used by various countries throughout the ages to create a unique flavor in their dishes.

Chinese Five Spice Powder: Chinese cooks typically use all the spices present in this powder to braise meat; creating the Chinese five spice powder ahead of time provides you with a time-saving shortcut! It's the basis of popular Chinese recipes, including five-spice chicken, char siu pork, and Peking duck.

Garam Masala Seasoning: Garam masala, which roughly translates to "hot spice mix" in Hindu, is used in many Indian recipes. The spices combine to create a sweet and savory mix commonly used to make curry and well-known classics like chicken tikka masala.

Jamaican Jerk Seasoning: In this sense, "jerk" originated in Jamaica and refers to a specific way of cooking and seasoning meat, vegetables, or fruit. Jerk chicken is one of the best-known Jamaican foods that has made its way to the United States. Jamaican jerk seasoning can help you achieve that famous "jerk" flavor when replicating Jamaican recipes. Tip: *Food and Wine Magazine* recommends adding 1 tablespoon of Chinese five spice powder as a secret ingredient to Jamaican jerk chicken to amp up the flavor.

Pumpkin Spice Mix: Fall has almost become synonymous with pumpkin spice. The popular flavor and scent is found everywhere, from the wildly popular pumpkin spice lattes, to pumpkin spice candles, to pumpkin spice hummus. The key to all of it is an easy-to-make blend of spices, which is where this pumpkin spice mix comes in. You can use it to add a festive flair to any recipe— sweet or savory.

Apple Pie Spice Mix: If you want apple pie flavor without the work of making an actual apple pie, this mix does the trick! Inspired by the taste of a freshly baked homemade apple pie, it combines key spices you can use to make anything taste like a pie. It's especially cozy sprinkled on top of oatmeal or apple sauce.

All spices can be stored in a glass jar away from heat and light.

CHINESE FIVE SPICE POWDER

6 whole star anise

1 1/2 whole cloves

1 cinnamon stick

2 tablespoons fennel seeds

2 teaspoons Sichuan peppercorns

1.　Grind all the spices together in a spice blender.

CURRY POWDER

2 tablespoons coriander

2 tablespoons cumin

1 1/2 tablespoons turmeric powder

2 teaspoons ground cardamom

2 teaspoons ground ginger

1 teaspoon dry mustard

1 teaspoon cinnamon powder

1 teaspoon cayenne pepper

1/2 teaspoon ground black pepper

1.　Combine all ingredients and use as needed.

GARAM MASALA SEASONING

1 tablespoon ground cumin

1 1/2 teaspoons ground coriander

1 1/2 teaspoons ground cardamom

1 1/2 teaspoons ground black pepper

1 teaspoon ground cinnamon

1 teaspoon red chili flakes

1/2 teaspoon ground cloves

1/2 teaspoon ground nutmeg

1.   Combine all ingredients and use as needed.

JAMAICAN JERK SEASONING

1 tablespoon onion powder

1 tablespoon garlic powder

1 tablespoon brown sugar or coconut sugar

1 tablespoon dried parsley

2 teaspoons ground ginger

2 teaspoons cayenne pepper

2 teaspoons smoked paprika

2 teaspoons salt

1 teaspoon allspice

1 teaspoon dried thyme

1 teaspoon black pepper

1/2 teaspoon red pepper flakes

1/2 teaspoon cumin

1/2 teaspoon nutmeg

1/2 teaspoon cinnamon

1.   Combine all ingredients and use as needed.

PUMPKIN SPICE MIX

4 teaspoons ground cinnamon

2 teaspoons ground ginger

1 teaspoon ground cloves

1/2 teaspoon ground nutmeg

1/2 teaspoon allspice

1. Combine all ingredients and use as needed.

APPLE PIE SPICE MIX

1 tablespoon ground cinnamon

1 teaspoon ground nutmeg

1 teaspoon allspice

1. Combine all ingredients and use as needed.

8. LEVEL UP YOUR BAKING

Baked goods taste delicious, but unfortunately, the combination of sugar and carbs typically spikes our blood sugar, resulting in brain fog and an eventual sugar crash. Here's where using cinnamon and alternative flours in your baked goods comes in.

Cinnamon can help manage blood sugar levels by regulating the glucose in your body.[16] Additionally, using flours that are higher in fiber and lower in carbohydrates allows the body to digest the food slower, stabilizing your blood sugar.[17] Some of these flours include popular gluten-free flours like spelt flour, almond flour, coconut flour, and garbanzo bean flour.

The recipes below are sweet without being overpoweringly sweet and are made with cinnamon and high-fiber alternative flours.

NUTRITION

BEAUTY

HEALTH

HOME

PALEO CINNAMON RAISIN BAGELS

1/2 cup cassava flour
1/4 cup almond flour
1/4 cup tapioca flour
1 cup arrowroot flour
1/4 cup maple syrup
1/4 cup ghee or butter
4 medium eggs + 1 medium egg (beaten)
1 tablespoon ground cinnamon, divided
1/2 cup raisins
1 teaspoon baking powder
1 teaspoon sea salt

1. Preheat the oven to 350°F and line a baking sheet with parchment paper.
2. Combine all of the ingredients—except for one medium egg (beaten), half of the cinnamon, and the raisins—in a large bowl or stand mixer.
3. Mix until the dough is smooth.
4. Gently fold in the rest of the cinnamon and raisins.
5. Separate the dough into six equal parts. Roll each part into a ball and shape it into a bagel by removing the center.
6. Fill a large saucepan half-full with water.
7. Bring the water to a boil. Turn the heat down slightly but keep the water boiling.
8. Drop one bagel at a time into the boiling water (using tongs is recommended).
9. Cook for one minute on each side or until the bagel floats to the top.
10. Place the boiled bagels on the baking sheet. Brush the egg wash on top.
11. Bake the bagels for about 30 minutes, or until the tops are golden brown.

NUTRITION

BEAUTY

HEALTH

HOME

GLUTEN-FREE BANANA BREAD

DRY INGREDIENTS:

3 scoops collagen powder
1/2 cup paleo or gluten-free flour mix
2 tablespoons coconut flour
2 tablespoons flaxseed meal
1 teaspoon cinnamon
1 teaspoon baking powder
1 teaspoon baking soda
Pinch of sea salt

WET INGREDIENTS:

4 ripe bananas
4 eggs
1/4 cup nut butter (natural is best)
2 tablespoons melted coconut oil
2 tablespoons ghee
1 teaspoon vanilla extract

MIX-INS:

1/2 cup walnuts, roughly chopped
1/3 cup dark chocolate chips or chunks (cacao nibs work too)

1. Preheat the oven to 375°F and grease a loaf pan.
2. Combine all dry ingredients in a small bowl.
3. In a large bowl, combine all wet ingredients.
4. Slowly fold the dry ingredients into the wet and use a fork to mix.
5. Gently fold in the walnuts and chocolate chips.
6. Pour the batter into the greased loaf pan and bake for 50 minutes to an hour.
7. Let cool and enjoy!

MAMA'S APPLE PIE

FOR THE CRUST:

3 cups almond flour

1 cup tapioca flour

12 tablespoons grass-fed butter (cold and cubed)

2 tablespoons coconut flour

2 tablespoons coconut sugar

1/2 teaspoon salt

1 large egg

FOR THE FILLING:

2.5 pounds apples, peeled, cored, and sliced

1/4 cup maple sugar

2 tablespoons maple syrup

2 tablespoons tapioca flour

2 tablespoons lemon juice

2 tablespoons coconut oil, melted

1 tablespoon vanilla extract

2 teaspoons cinnamon

1/4 teaspoon nutmeg

1/4 teaspoon allspice

1/4 teaspoon ground ginger

1. Combine the dry crust ingredients in a food processor until they form a coarse mixture.
2. Whisk the egg and add to the dry ingredients.
3. Using your hands, mix together so it forms a dough.
4. Separate the dough into two equal parts and press into flat circles.
5. Wrap the dough in plastic wrap and chill in the refrigerator for at least an hour (however, overnight is recommended).
6. Preheat the oven to 425°F.

NUTRITION

BEAUTY

HEALTH

HOME

7. Place one of the dough circles in between two pieces of parchment paper (or silicone baking mats) and roll it out until it forms a circle about three inches larger in diameter than your pie dish.

8. Lay the dough in the pie dish and press it down gently. Put the dish in the freezer.

9. Combine the filling ingredients in a large bowl and toss until the apples are evenly coated.

10. Take the pie crust out of the freezer and fill it with the apples (try not to add the liquid).

11. Repeat the same rolling process between the parchment paper with the second circle of dough.

12. Remove the paper and slice the dough into thin strips. Carefully lay the strips in a crisscross lattice style on top of the pie.

13. Bake the pie for 10 minutes.

14. Lower the temperature to 375°F and bake for another 30–40 minutes, until the crust is golden brown.

15. Let cool and enjoy!

FEEL-GOOD GLUTEN-FREE CINNAMON ROLLS

FOR THE DOUGH:

1 organic, free-range egg
1 teaspoon pure vanilla extract
2 tablespoons chai concentrate
3 tablespoons coconut oil, melted
1 tablespoon agave syrup or raw honey
1 1/2 cups cassava flour
1/2 cup almond flour
2 scoops collagen powder
1 teaspoon baking soda

1 teaspoon cinnamon
2 tablespoons golden flaxseed meal
Pinch of organic sea salt

FOR THE FILLING:

3 tablespoons organic pumpkin puree
1 tablespoon cinnamon
1/4 cup organic walnuts or pecans, finely chopped
4 pitted Medjool dates, soaked and finely chopped
1 tablespoon raw honey

FOR THE TOPPING:

Raw almond butter or honey, for drizzling

1. Mix the wet ingredients for the dough and whisk lightly until combined.
2. In a separate bowl, combine the dry ingredients for the dough.
3. Slowly fold the dry ingredients into the wet and then use your hands to combine. If not sticking together properly, add more melted coconut oil and a bit of warm water.
4. Place the dough on a piece of wax paper. Place another piece of wax paper on top and roll out the dough into a thin, flat sheet.
5. Remove the top piece of wax paper.
6. Spread the dough with the pumpkin puree first and then add the cinnamon, nuts, and dates; top with a generous drizzle of honey.
7. Use the bottom piece of wax paper to roll the dough into a log and place in the freezer for 15 minutes to harden.
8. Preheat the oven to 355°F and grease a baking sheet.
9. Take the dough out of the freezer and remove the wax paper. Cut the dough into rounds and place on the greased baking pan.

BEAUTY

HEALTH

HOME

10. Bake for about 15 minutes or until golden.
11. Top with a drizzle of nut butter or honey, or create your own paleo-friendly cinnamon roll glaze with coconut cream and honey!

9. FLAVOR MEAT

Centuries ago, cinnamon was used to preserve meat because it has antibacterial properties.[18] These days, although the spice is no longer needed for preservation, the subtle sweetness of the spice helps bring out the flavor of the meat.[19]

APPLE PIE PORK CHOPS

FOR THE PORK:
2 sprigs fresh rosemary
1 teaspoon cinnamon
1 teaspoon smoked paprika
1/2 teaspoon nutmeg
Pinch of sea salt
2 bone-in pork chops
1 tablespoon coconut oil

FOR THE APPLES:
1/2 tablespoon coconut oil
2 apples, cored and sliced
1 small red onion, sliced
4 ounces bone broth
1 tablespoon fresh sage, roughly chopped
1 tablespoon maple syrup
1 teaspoon cinnamon
1 teaspoon ground ginger

NUTRITION

BEAUTY

HEALTH

HOME

1 teaspoon spicy brown mustard
Sea salt
Freshly ground black pepper

1. Combine the spices for the pork and rub on both sides of the pork chop.
2. Heat a cast-iron skillet or large pan over high heat. Add the coconut oil when the skillet is hot and lower the heat to medium high.
3. Add the pork chops and brown for three minutes on each side.
4. Remove the pork chops from the skillet/pan and set aside.
5. Add the coconut oil to the skillet/pan, followed by the apples and onions. Allow them to brown and soften slightly.
6. Add the rest of the ingredients for the apples and stir to combine.
7. Add the pork chops and simmer over medium heat until they are fully cooked (2–3 minutes).
8. Remove from the heat and enjoy!

PALEO PUMPKIN CHILI
1 1/2 tablespoons avocado oil
2 pounds ground turkey or beef (you can also do half and half)
1 small red onion, diced
1 bell pepper, diced
28 ounces fire-roasted tomatoes
16 ounces canned pumpkin
8 ounces bone broth
1 1/2 tablespoons chili powder
1 tablespoon cacao powder
1 1/2 teaspoons garlic powder
1 1/2 teaspoons cinnamon
1 1/2 teaspoons cumin
1/2 teaspoon nutmeg

NUTRITION

BEAUTY

HEALTH

HOME

1/2 teaspoon smoked paprika (regular paprika works too)
1/2 teaspoon cayenne powder
Sea salt, to taste
Freshly ground black pepper, to taste
Dairy-free, plain Greek yogurt or sour cream, for topping
Avocado, diced, for topping
Jalapeño, sliced, for topping

1. Heat a large pan over high heat. Add avocado oil when hot.

2. Add the ground meat to brown.

3. Once the meat is browned, add the onions and peppers and cook for 2 minutes.

4. Heat a large pot over medium-high heat and add the meat, onions, and peppers from the pan.

5. Pour in the rest of the ingredients and stir to combine.

6. Bring the chili to a boil, then lower the heat to a simmer. Simmer for 30 minutes. If you like a thinner chili, you can add a little more bone broth at the halfway point.

7. Remove from the heat and serve. You can top with plain Greek yogurt or sour cream, avocados, and/or jalapeños if desired.

10. COOK FOOD FROM AROUND THE WORLD

Cinnamon has been used in cuisines around the world for centuries, ranging from sweet (like Mexican hot chocolate) to savory (like Indian curry). It's a versatile spice that allows you to cook food from around the world right in your own kitchen!

CHINESE CHILI OIL

3 tablespoons toasted white sesame seeds

3/4 cup crushed red pepper flakes (I recommend Sichuan chili flakes)

1 teaspoon salt

1 1/2 cups grapeseed oil

5 whole star anise

1 cinnamon stick

2 bay leaves

3 tablespoons Sichuan peppercorns

1 tablespoon fresh ginger, minced

1. Mix the sesame seeds, red pepper flakes, and salt in a bowl; set aside.

2. Mix the oil, star anise, cinnamon stick, bay leaves, peppercorns, and ginger in a small saucepan and set over medium-high heat.

3. Once you see the oil bubble, turn the heat down to low. You want to avoid burning the oil and spices, so if you have a thermometer, make sure the temperature is between 200°F and 225°F.

4. Simmer the oil for 30 minutes. It should be slightly bubbling the whole time; adjust the heat slightly if it's not.

5. Remove from the heat and strain the mixture over the bowl with the sesame seeds, red pepper flakes, and salt.

6. Stir well and let cool. Transfer to a jar and store in the refrigerator for up to three months.

BEAUTY

HEALTH

HOME

MOROCCAN TURMERIC CAULIFLOWER SOUP

1 head cauliflower
4 medium garlic cloves, peeled
1 teaspoon salt
4 tablespoons extra virgin olive oil, divided
1 large yellow onion, diced
1 carrot, peeled and diced
4 cups bone broth or vegetable broth
1 teaspoon cumin
1 teaspoon coriander
1 teaspoon ground ginger
1 teaspoon turmeric
1 teaspoon cinnamon
1 teaspoon paprika
1 teaspoon black pepper
Sliced green onion, for garnish

1. Preheat the oven to 375°F and line a baking sheet with parchment paper.
2. Chop the cauliflower into small florets.
3. Toss together the cauliflower, garlic, salt, and two tablespoons of olive oil.
4. Place the cauliflower on the lined baking sheet and roast for 40 minutes.
5. Heat two tablespoons of olive oil in a large pot over medium-high heat.
6. Add the onion and carrot and sauté until the carrots are softer and the onion is translucent (about 3 minutes).
7. Add the broth and spices. Simmer for 10 minutes.
8. Add the cauliflower when it's done roasting and use a blender to puree the soup.
9. Serve immediately and top with sliced green onions if desired.

EASY AND FLAVORFUL INDIAN CURRY

2 tablespoons coconut oil or ghee, divided

1 1/2 pounds lamb, chopped into cubes

1/2 tablespoon fresh garlic, minced

1/2 tablespoon fresh ginger, minced

4 teaspoons yellow curry powder

2 teaspoons turmeric

1 teaspoon ground cumin

1 teaspoon garam masala

1 teaspoon cayenne powder

2 teaspoons salt

2 bay leaves

2 whole cloves

1 cinnamon stick

1/2 cup onion, diced

14 ounces full-fat coconut milk

1 1/2 cups crushed tomatoes

1 tablespoon fresh cilantro, minced

Basmati rice or cauliflower rice, for serving

Naan, for serving

1. Heat one tablespoon of the coconut oil or ghee in a large pan on medium-high heat.

2. Brown the lamb cubes in the pan for 2–3 minutes, or until browned on both sides. Pour onto a plate and set aside.

3. Add the second tablespoon of coconut oil or ghee to the pan and lower the heat to medium.

4. Add all the spices and the onion. Cook until the onion is translucent.

5. Add the coconut milk and tomatoes and continue cooking. When the curry comes to a boil (you may have to increase the heat to do so), allow to boil for 3 minutes.

6. Turn the heat to low and simmer for 15 minutes while covered.

7. Add the lamb and the cilantro. Simmer uncovered for another 5 minutes or until the lamb is cooked through.

8. Serve with rice of choice and/or naan and enjoy!

....

11. MAKE DESSERTS EXTRA SWEET

One of the most commonly used spices in desserts is cinnamon. This spice naturally boosts the sweetness of your desserts without adding any sugar. This innate sweetness allows you to lessen the amount of added sugar in your desserts if you're looking to cut back on your sugar intake.

You can do more with cinnamon than simply make apple pie, however. It's been used in a variety of cuisines for centuries, from the age-old, multicultural rice pudding to the fairly recent American "nice" cream.

CHOCOLATE CINNAMON "NICE" CREAM

4 ripe bananas, sliced and frozen
3 tablespoons cacao powder
2 tablespoons sunflower seed butter
1 tablespoon unsweetened coconut milk
1 teaspoon ground cinnamon
1 teaspoon vanilla extract
Pinch of sea salt

1. Combine all ingredients in a food processor or high-speed blender and pulse until smooth. Add more coconut milk if necessary to help blend the bananas.

2. Serve immediately and enjoy!

DAIRY-FREE CINNAMON RICE PUDDING

3 cups unsweetened macadamia, hemp, or flax milk (these are the creamiest)

1/2 cup short-grain brown rice (you can use white rice as well—increase to 3/4 cup if you do)

1/2 cup coconut cream

1/2 cup raisins

1/4 cup maple syrup

2 teaspoons ground cinnamon

1 teaspoon vanilla extract

1 teaspoon ground cardamom (optional)

1 teaspoon orange zest

1/2 teaspoon ground nutmeg

Pinch of salt, to taste

Pistachios, shelled, for topping

1. Combine ingredients in a large pot and cook on medium heat until it comes to a boil.
2. Reduce the heat to low and simmer for 20 minutes. Stir occasionally so the rice doesn't stick to the bottom.
3. Taste and add more sweeteners or spices if desired.
4. Serve warm and top with pistachios if desired, or chill in the fridge and top with pistachios right before serving.

CRAZY CANDIED BACON

6 strips bacon (thick but not thick-cut)

2 tablespoons maple syrup

1 tablespoon coconut sugar

1 teaspoon cinnamon

1 teaspoon cayenne pepper

1. Preheat the oven to 400°F.
2. Line a baking sheet with aluminum foil and place a wire rack on top. Spread the bacon on top of the wire rack.
3. Cook the bacon for 10 minutes.

NUTRITION

BEAUTY

HEALTH

HOME

4. Remove the bacon from the oven and lower the heat to 350°F.

5. Blot the bacon with a paper towel.

6. Combine the maple syrup and spices in a large glass pan. Cover one side of each bacon slice in the spiced maple syrup.

7. Cook the bacon for 10 minutes in the oven, maple-syrup side up.

8. Remove from the oven, blot, and then cover the second side with maple syrup.

9. Cook the bacon for another 10 minutes in the oven, fresh maple-syrup side up.

10. Remove the pan from the oven and let it cool for 10–20 minutes before enjoying.

12. POWER UP YOUR SNACKS

Cinnamon is an incredible spice to add to snacks for kids and adults alike. It helps enhance cognition, making it perfect for an after-school homework snack or an afternoon workday snack.[20]

SWEET CINNAMON ALMONDS

1 cup almonds

1/8 cup maple syrup

1 tablespoon coconut oil

1 teaspoon cinnamon

1 teaspoon vanilla extract

NUTRITION

BEAUTY

HEALTH

HOME

Pinch of pink Himalayan salt

1. Preheat the oven to 325°F.
2. Line a baking sheet with parchment paper or a nonstick silicone baking mat.
3. Pour the almonds on top of the prepared baking sheet and roast for 10 minutes.
4. Combine maple syrup, coconut oil, cinnamon, and vanilla extract in a pan. Bring to a boil, then lower to medium-low heat.
5. Add the almonds and simmer, stirring frequently, until the maple syrup starts to evaporate (about 3–5 minutes).
6. Lay the nuts out flat on the lined baking sheet.
7. Sprinkle salt on top and allow to cool before eating or storing.

CINNAMON PLANTAIN CHIPS

1 green plantain
1 tablespoon melted coconut oil
1 teaspoon cinnamon
1/2 teaspoon pink Himalayan salt

1. Preheat the oven to 350°F.
2. Line a baking sheet with parchment paper or a nonstick silicone baking mat.
3. Cut off the ends of the plantain. Then cut three shallow scores in the skin so the knife cuts through the skin but not into the flesh. Peel the skin off.
4. Slice the plantain into 1/4-inch thick slices.
5. In a small bowl, toss the plantain chips, coconut oil, cinnamon, and sea salt.
6. Spread the plantain chips in a thin layer on the baking sheet and bake for 25 minutes, until crisp and crunchy.

NUTRITION

BEAUTY

HEALTH

HOME

NUTRITION

BEAUTY

HEALTH

HOME

FRUIT SALSA WITH CINNAMON PITA CHIPS

FOR THE FRUIT SALSA:

1 cup strawberries, chopped

1 kiwi, diced

1 nectarine, diced

4 ounces raspberries

4 ounces blueberries

4 ounces blackberries

2 tablespoons honey

1 tablespoon lemon juice

FOR THE PITA CHIPS:

4 grain-free tortillas (Siete Foods has great ones!)

1 tablespoon coconut oil, melted

1 tablespoon coconut sugar

1/2 teaspoon cinnamon

1. Preheat the oven to 350°F and line a baking sheet with parchment paper.
2. Combine all fruit salsa ingredients together and store in an airtight container until use.
3. Cut the tortillas into triangles (imagine you're cutting a pizza).
4. Brush the melted coconut oil on both sides of each chip.
5. Mix the coconut sugar and cinnamon together well. Sprinkle on both sides of each chip.
6. Spread the chips out on the prepared baking sheet and bake for 10 minutes.
7. Let cool completely before serving with the fruit salsa.

NO-ADDED-SUGAR APPLESAUCE

2 tablespoons ghee or coconut oil

3 pounds apples, peeled, cored, and thickly chopped

1/4 cup water
1 teaspoon lemon juice
1 teaspoon ground cinnamon
1 teaspoon vanilla extract
1/2 teaspoon nutmeg
1 whole star anise

1. Heat coconut oil or ghee in a large pot over high heat.
2. Add all ingredients to the pot and simmer on low heat for 45 minutes to an hour. Stir occasionally—every 15 minutes or so.
3. Taste the mixture and add more cinnamon if desired. The texture of the apples should be soft.
4. Let cool and store in a container in the fridge for up to a week.

IRRESISTIBLE APPLE CHIPS

2 pounds apples
1 tablespoon cinnamon

1. Core the apples and slice into thin rounds.
2. Toss the apple slices with the cinnamon, dehydrate using a food dehydrator or oven, and store for up to two weeks.

USING A FOOD DEHYDRATOR:

Turn the dehydrator to 135°F and dehydrate the apples for 6 hours, or until they are no longer moist. (If your dehydrator has specific instructions for dehydrating fruit, you can follow those instead.)

USING AN OVEN:

Preheat the oven to 200°F and line a baking sheet with parchment paper. Lay the cinnamon-coated apple slices on top of the baking sheet, ensuring there is no overlap. Bake the apples for 1 hour, then flip them and allow to bake for another 1 to 2 hours until the chips are no longer moist.

NUTRITION

BEAUTY

HEALTH

HOME

13. COZY UP YOUR BREAKFAST

Eating cinnamon for breakfast helps you start your day off strong! Not only does it make your entire breakfast cozy and sweet, but it also gives you a wonderful boost of health benefits: cinnamon has been shown to reduce inflammation, lower blood sugar, and be packed with antioxidants that fight free radicals (cell-damaging molecules) in your body.[21] It also has memory-boosting properties, which help you head off to work or school with a clear head.[22]

BREAKFAST CINNAMON SWEET POTATOES

1 sweet potato
Yogurt, to taste
Blueberries, to taste
Nut Butter, to taste
Granola, to taste
Cinnamon, to taste

1. Preheat the oven to 375°F.
2. Wash the sweet potato, place on a baking sheet, and bake for an hour, or until the inside is soft.
3. Cut the potato in half and stuff with yogurt, blueberries, nut butter, and granola.
4. Top with a sprinkle of cinnamon and enjoy!

CINNAMON 'N' OATMEAL

FOR THE OATMEAL:
1/3 cup riced cauliflower
1/3 cup milk of choice
1 tablespoon flaxseed meal
1 tablespoon chia seeds
1 tablespoon hemp hearts
1 tablespoon almond flour
1 scoop collagen powder (optional)
1/2 banana
1 teaspoon cinnamon
1 teaspoon vanilla extract

FOR THE TOPPINGS:
Fresh blueberries, to taste
Honey, to taste
Walnuts, to taste
Nut butter, to taste

1. In a small pot, combine all ingredients except the vanilla extract and toppings.
2. Simmer on low heat, stirring occasionally, until the cauliflower and banana are soft and cooked through. You may need to add more milk.
3. Add in the vanilla extract and stir to combine. Remove from the heat and top as desired.

USING A MICROWAVE:
You can put all ingredients, minus the toppings, in a microwave-safe bowl and microwave for 2–3 minutes. Once warm, add your toppings and enjoy!

NOT-YOUR-DIET BREAKFAST BROILED GRAPEFRUIT

FOR THE GRAPEFRUIT:

1 grapefruit

2 tablespoons honey

1/2 teaspoon cinnamon

1/2 teaspoon cayenne

1/2 teaspoon ground ginger

FOR THE TOPPINGS:

Yogurt, to taste

Walnuts, to taste

Fresh fruit, to taste

1. Cut the ends off the grapefruit, so it doesn't roll, and then cut it in half.
2. Combine the honey and spices. Spread the paste on both halves of the grapefruit.
3. Broil the grapefruit for 5–8 minutes, or until golden brown on top.
4. Top with yogurt, walnuts, and fruit; enjoy!

CINNAMON COFFEE SMOOTHIE

6 ounces nut milk

6 ounces cold brew

1/2 ripe banana, frozen (you can use fresh as well, but you may need to add a few ice cubes)

1/4 cup frozen riced cauliflower

1 tablespoon almond butter

1 tablespoon flaxseed meal

1 tablespoon hemp hearts

1 teaspoon cinnamon

1 teaspoon vanilla extract

1-2 pitted dates (optional)

1. Combine all ingredients in a high-speed blender.
2. Blend until creamy. You may need to add more liquid to loosen up the blender.
3. Pour into a cup and enjoy!

CINNAMON BREAKFAST TOAST

2 slices of bread
Butter or vegan butter, to taste
Honey, to taste
Cinnamon, to taste

1. Toast the bread.
2. Spread butter thickly over each slice of toast.
3. Drizzle the honey and liberally sprinkle the cinnamon on top.
4. Enjoy!

14. PICKLE FOOD

Pickling food has actually been around for about four thousand years as a way to preserve food for later months and rations on long journeys.[23] These days, we no longer have to preserve food out of necessity, but pickling remains a delicious way to add extra veggies to our diet. There are two versions of pickling:

Quick pickling: This uses vinegar to preserve food by immersion in an acidic solution.

Fermentation: This is the result of a chemical reaction between a food's sugar and natural bacteria.

Cinnamon is especially helpful in pickling food because it has antimicrobial properties.[24] Although the process of sterilizing the jars and pickling should kill any unwanted bacteria, adding cinnamon to the pickles while making them can help prevent any additional bacteria from forming. The recipe below is for quick pickling—you only need 48 hours for the cucumbers to pickle.

QUICK HOMEMADE PICKLES

Baby cucumbers (or regular, but you may have to slice them thinner)
2 bay leaves
1 cinnamon stick
1/2 teaspoon nutmeg
1/2 teaspoon yellow mustard seeds
1/2 teaspoon paprika
1 cup apple cider vinegar
1 cup water
1/2 cup sugar
Pinch of sea salt

1. Cut the cucumbers in half lengthwise and trim off the ends.
2. Sterilize a large glass jar by using boiling water.
3. Rinse the inside of the jar with fresh boiling water.
4. Add all spices to the jar.
5. Add the cucumbers to the jar. Pack them as tightly as you can.
6. Combine the vinegar, water, sugar, and salt in a pan. Bring the brine to a boil.
7. Pour the brine into the jar until there is half an inch of space left at the top.
8. Tap the jar gently against the counter to remove any air bubbles. Add more brine if necessary.
9. Put the lid on the jar and seal tightly.
10. Let the jar cool at room temperature.
11. Refrigerate for 48 hours before eating.
12. Store in the fridge for up to a week.

15. FLAVOR YOUR VEGGIES

Cinnamon may seem intuitive in baked goods and breakfast because it's a typically sweet spice, but it works just as well in vegetable dishes. It creates a sweet-and-salty combo that's hard to resist! It makes eating your veggies easier and tastier.

MOROCCAN-STYLE CINNAMON SPICED CARROTS

SALAD VERSION

FOR THE SALAD:

1/4 cup raisins (regular or golden)
1/2 pound carrots
1/2 bunch cilantro, plus more for topping

FOR THE DRESSING:

2 tablespoons tahini
1 tablespoon olive oil
1 tablespoon honey or maple syrup
1 teaspoon lemon juice
1 teaspoon ground cinnamon
1/2 teaspoon cayenne
1/2 teaspoon turmeric
Large pinch of sea salt
Freshly ground black pepper, to taste

1. Soak the raisins in a bowl of water; this will help rehydrate them.
2. Wash and scrub carrots. Remove greens if present.

3. Grate carrots roughly until they're shredded into thin, long slices (you can also buy them preshredded). Alternatively, you can grate them into wider ribbons for a different aesthetic.

4. Wash the cilantro before rolling it into a bundle and roughly chopping. This will help preserve the taste.

5. In a small bowl, combine all ingredients for the dressing. Whisk thoroughly with a fork.

6. Drain the raisins and place them, the shredded carrots, and the cilantro in a large bowl.

7. Pour the dressing on top and toss.

8. Grind fresh black pepper on top.

9. Garnish with more cilantro if desired and enjoy!

ROASTED VERSION

1 pound carrots
1 tablespoon honey or maple syrup
2 tablespoons avocado oil or coconut oil
1 teaspoon smoked paprika
1 teaspoon cumin
1 teaspoon turmeric powder
1/2 teaspoon ground ginger
1/2 teaspoon ground cinnamon
1/2 teaspoon cayenne powder
Large pinch of sea salt
Black pepper, freshly ground, to taste
1/4 cup raisins (regular or golden)
Cilantro, for garnish
Tahini, to taste (optional)

1. Preheat the oven to 375°F.

2. Scrub and wash carrots. Remove greens if present.

3. Cut the carrots into diagonal 1 1/2–inch pieces and place in a large baking pan.

4. In a separate bowl, combine the honey or maple syrup, avocado or coconut oil, and seasonings. Whisk with a fork until thoroughly combined.

5. Pour the mixture over the carrots and toss to coat evenly.

6. Roast the carrots for 20 minutes.

7. While the carrots are roasting, soak the raisins in water; this will help rehydrate them.

8. Drain raisins after 20 minutes. Sprinkle them on top of the carrots and return to the oven for another 5 minutes.

9. Remove the carrots from the oven. Grind black pepper on top and garnish with cilantro. They taste great with a drizzle of tahini as well!

UPGRADED ANTS ON A LOG

3 stalks celery
3–6 tablespoons almond butter
Cinnamon, to taste
Sea salt, to taste
1/4 cup goji berries or dried cranberries
Honey, for drizzling (optional)

1. Wash the celery and trim the ends. Cut into 2- to 3-inch-long sections and pat dry.

2. Spread almond butter in the hollow part of each celery segment.

3. Sprinkle cinnamon and sea salt on top.

4. Place goji berries or dried cranberries in the hollows of the celery and press in gently.

5. Drizzle honey on top if desired and enjoy!

NUTRITION

FALL BALSAMIC CINNAMON ROASTED VEGGIES

1 pound fall vegetables: Brussels sprouts, sweet potatoes, squash, turnips, etc.

2 tablespoons balsamic vinegar

2 tablespoons extra virgin olive oil

1 tablespoon honey

1 teaspoon Dijon mustard

1 teaspoon cinnamon

1/2 teaspoon smoked paprika

Large pinch of sea salt

2 sprigs rosemary

1. Preheat the oven to 375°F.
2. Wash and scrub the vegetables. Dice them into bite-sized pieces and pat dry before placing them on a large baking pan.
3. Combine the vinegar, olive oil, honey, Dijon mustard, cinnamon, paprika, and sea salt in a bowl and whisk thoroughly.
4. Pour the dressing over the veggies and toss to coat evenly.
5. Bake for 30 minutes.
6. Add rosemary to the top and bake for another 10–15 minutes.
7. Remove from the oven and enjoy!

BEAUTY

HEALTH

16. INFUSE FOODS

Infusing oils and spirits is an easy way to create a fancier, more unique experience and take your bottle of olive oil or whiskey from ordinary to extraordinary! All you need is some cinnamon, liquid of choice, and time.

Infusing is simply steeping an ingredient in a liquid until the liquid has absorbed the ingredient's taste.[25] Theoretically, by this definition, tea and coffee are infusions, but we'll get fancier than

HOME

that. The two recipes below help you infuse two common liquids—oil and alcohol. They make for beautiful gifts, as well as a simple way to spice up your everyday cooking and drinking.

CINNAMON INFUSED OLIVE OIL

2 cups pure olive oil

1/2 cup ground cinnamon

1. Heat olive oil in a large pan over medium to high heat.
2. Once the oil is warm, add cinnamon and stir to combine.
3. Lower heat to a simmer and continue cooking for about 3 minutes.
4. Remove from the heat and strain through a coffee filter to remove as much of the cinnamon as possible.
5. Store in a sterilized glass bottle (ideally a dark bottle so it's unaffected by sunlight) for up to a month.

CINNAMON INFUSED ALCOHOL

2 cups spirit of choice (I recommend vodka, whiskey, or bourbon)

2 cinnamon sticks

1. Place cinnamon sticks in a large Mason jar.
2. Pour the alcohol in.
3. Seal tightly and leave for up to two weeks. Taste it every few days—once it gets to your desired spice level, pour into a clean glass jar and enjoy! You can give this as a gift, make this into cocktails, or simply sip on its own over ice.

NUTRITION

BEAUTY

HEALTH

HOME

CHAPTER 2

FOR THE BEAUTY LOVER IN YOU

17. CIRCULATION- BOOSTING BODY OIL

In the Bible, cinnamon was used in the holy anointing oil (Exodus 30: 23–14), which was made with myrrh, cinnamon, and olive oil. While you can use a version of this blend to make your own anointing oil if you're so inclined, this oil serves best as a quick-absorbing body oil after your shower or as a warming massage oil.

People typically think of massages as something you have to go to the spa for, but you can perform a massage right at home—either on yourself or with the help of a partner. Whether it's a head and scalp, hand and foot, back, or full-body massage, the benefits are numerous. It can help with anxiety and depression,[1] boost your immune system, and lower your stress levels.[2]

Many masseuses like using coconut oil or lotion to lubricate the skin as they massage it, but this homemade version provides extra benefits: the jojoba and olive oils are less likely to clog your skin and are hydrating and quick-absorbing, so you won't feel greasy or sticky afterward.

Cinnamon plays an important part in the warming process—it's commonly known as a "warming spice" that can improve blood flow.[3] Combined with other essential oils that also boost circulation, not only does this body oil smell great, but it will prepare your muscles for massage or keep you warm long after you've finished your shower.

WARMING CINNAMON BODY OIL

5 drops clove essential oil
15 drops cinnamon essential oil
5 drops ginger essential oil
10 drops vanilla essential oil
5 drops sandalwood essential oil
1/4 cup jojoba oil
1/4 cup olive oil
10 milliliters CBD oil (optional)

1. Combine all ingredients in a squeeze bottle and shake well. Use as needed.

18. FACE MASK

Not only are face masks a great way to relax and enjoy some self-care time, but they are also a way to give your skin powerful ingredients that it doesn't typically get in your normal skincare routine. Masks nowadays are made with anything from snail mucus (yes, really) to the classic green clay. However, you don't need fancy ingredients to have an effective face mask—you can create a potent face mask with products you already have in your pantry.

One of the benefits of DIY masks is you're able to control exactly what goes into them. All the ingredients in this honey cinnamon mask are ones you can eat—that's how you know it's safe for your skin to absorb! The combination of cinnamon and honey is a powerful one—while both have antibacterial effects, once combined, the two ingredients are even more effective against acne-causing bacteria (*Propionibacterium acnes* and *Staphylococcus epidermidis*).[4] Extra benefits of cinnamon include reducing fine lines by boosting blood circulation and relieving eczema.[5]

Honey has additional exfoliating properties; it naturally contains glycolic acid, which is a chemical exfoliant that gets rid of your dead skin cells without physically scrubbing them off. Additionally, honey keeps your skin moisturized by absorbing moisture from the environment and locking it underneath your skin.

ACNE-FIGHTING CINNAMON HONEY MASK

2 tablespoons honey (I recommend manuka honey)

1 teaspoon cinnamon

1. Combine ingredients together to form a paste.
2. Spread all over your face and leave on for 10–15 minutes.
3. Rinse off with warm water and pat dry or let air dry.
4. Follow skincare routine as usual.

19. ACNE SPOT TREATMENT

Having healthy and clear skin is something people of all ages aim for. It has long been a symbol of physical health in our society and can boost self-confidence and emotional well-being in women (who can think of flawless skin as the canvas for any makeup they apply) and men alike.[6]

Beyond the emotional benefits of clear skin, it's important to take care of your skin for many other reasons, including that it's your body's largest organ! Underlying health issues or allergic reactions can present themselves on your skin, meaning acne, rosacea, or other skin issues may be an indicator of a bigger environmental or health problem. If you find yourself with persistent acne, try taking a look at your diet and the products you are using in your home and on your body; seeing if you have any other symptoms, like fatigue, moodiness, or weight gain; and perhaps even visiting a dermatologist, traditional Chinese medicine doctor, or naturopath.

To recap: While there are a multitude of triggers for acne—including diet, skincare products, hormones, and your natural skin type—we *can* treat the actual spots the same, with the help of cinnamon. Acne is caused by the inflammation of hair follicles and their subsequent clogging of sebaceous (oil-producing) glands in the skin.[7] Thus, cinnamon is effective at treating acne spots because of its anti-inflammatory properties—a little cinnamon can help your spots look less red and raised. When combined with raw honey and tea tree oil, which both have antibacterial benefits, you create a potent homemade spot treatment you can use anytime you need.

QUICK ACNE SPOT TREATMENT

1 teaspoon cinnamon powder
3 teaspoons raw, local honey
1 drop tea tree oil

1. Combine all the ingredients to form a paste.
2. Spread the mixture on the desired spots.
3. Leave on for 15–30 minutes and wash off with warm water.
4. Follow with your regular skincare routine.

Note: It's recommended that you test homemade treatments on your neck or arm first to check for any potential reactions or sensitivities.

Note: Spot treatments are designed to help existing acne disappear quicker; they will not prevent more acne from forming.

20. HAIR LIGHTENER

Cinnamon and honey naturally contain peroxide, an agent that lightens hair.[8] Unlike store-bought hair dyes, using a cinnamon-based hair dye won't strip your hair of its natural oils (or its natural healthy shine!). In fact, cinnamon—combined with the hydrating properties of the natural ingredients in this hair dye—will help you get sun-kissed strands *and* hydrate your hair. Bonus: It smells great as well.

CINNAMON HAIR-LIGHTENING MASK

2 tablespoons lemon juice
1 tablespoon cinnamon
1 tablespoon olive oil or melted coconut oil
1 tablespoon natural honey

FOR A BLONDER COLOR:

5 bags chamomile tea, steeped

FOR A REDDER COLOR:

6-10 tablespoons henna

1. Mix all the ingredients until they form a mask-like paste. Add more olive oil if the mask is too thick.
2. Coat hair evenly with the mask.
3. Put hair in a high bun and leave on for at least 2 hours. Cover with a shower cap if possible. You can even leave this mask on overnight; just be sure to cover your pillow with a towel to keep it clean!

NUTRITION

BEAUTY

HEALTH

HOME

4. Wash out with your regular shampoo and conditioner. It may take two shampoos to get all of the mask out of your hair.
5. Let hair dry naturally.

21. HAIR GROWTH STIMULATOR

Thick, luscious hair is typically equated with good health and beauty. However, hair thinning and hair loss is a common problem as we age. According to the North American Hair Research Society, half of women experience some hair loss by the time they hit fifty.[9] In addition, women who were post-menopause have been shown to have lower hair density (less hair on the scalp) and slower rates of hair growth.[10] So how do we combat this?

Cinnamon essential oil can help! In an Indonesian study, cinnamon essential oil was proven to increase hair follicle length and diameter as effectively as minoxidil, a drug commonly used to stimulate hair growth and slow balding in both men and women.[11]

To boost your hair hydration and stimulate hair growth, you can use a conditioning oil. The recipe below combines certain botanicals that have been reported to stimulate hair growth with cinnamon essential oil for a fragrant hair-boosting treatment.[12]

HAIR-BOOSTING CONDITIONING OIL

1/4 cup almond oil
1/4 cup olive oil
5 drops cinnamon essential oil
1 teaspoon cayenne powder

1. Combine all ingredients in a dropper bottle.
2. Use one dropperful in wet or dry hair. Start by massaging into your scalp, then continue by bringing the oil all the way down to the ends.
3. Leave it in for at least 30 minutes, but overnight is recommended.
4. Shampoo out the next day as usual.

22. LIP EXFOLIANT

Nobody likes the feeling of dry, chapped lips. It's especially common in the cold winter months—harsh winds, cold temperatures, and dry air all take a toll on our bodies and strip the moisture from our skin.

Exfoliation helps remove the dead skin from your lips, but that can also leave your skin dry if you don't properly moisturize afterward or use a high-quality exfoliant. The hydrating yet effective combination of the ingredients in this homemade lip scrub will help you get rid of all the dead, flaky skin on your lips while providing your lips with much-needed hydration. Cinnamon not only provides a cozy scent and delicious taste to this lip scrub (while it is edible, we *don't* recommend eating it!), it also helps boost circulation in your lips, leading to a plumping effect.[13]

CINNAMON-SUGAR LIP SCRUB

4 tablespoons organic brown sugar
1 tablespoon raw honey
1 tablespoon extra virgin olive oil, avocado oil, or vitamin E oil
1 teaspoon organic ground cinnamon
1 drop vanilla essential oil (optional)

1. Combine all ingredients in a bowl and mix thoroughly.
2. Pour into a glass container for storage (you can also use an old lip balm pot that you've cleaned and washed).
3. Apply a small amount to your lips and rub gently in small circles.
4. Rinse off with warm water and pat dry.
5. Follow with a heavy-duty lip balm to keep your newly soft lips nice and moisturized.

23. DRY SKIN SCRUB

For some, itchy, peeling, dry skin (also known as xerosis) is a common ailment in the cold winter months. The wind, indoor heating systems, long hot showers, and drops in temperature can all affect our skin's ability to retain moisture, resulting in dry skin.

For others, dry skin is a year-round problem. As we age, our skin starts to lose its ability to retain moisture effectively, making dry skin more prevalent.[14] Fortunately, most dry skin can be remedied with simple solutions.

Hydration starts from the inside out, so start by increasing your water intake. Then you can adjust your environment—take warm (rather than hot) showers and use a humidifier in your house, especially in the winter. Finally, oil-based products will help lock in moisture better than water-based products. The sugar scrub below has coconut oil to hydrate you while you're in the shower, coffee grounds and cinnamon to increase circulation and provide scent, and honey to help keep your skin looking young.[15]

Gentle exfoliation is important to maintain smooth and supple skin—it helps scrub off the dry skin cells and reveal the new skin underneath. Be sure to moisturize with a hydrating cream, lotion, or oil after you get out of the shower to protect your newly exfoliated skin!

SWEET CINNAMON-SUGAR SCRUB

1 cup coconut oil, melted
2/3 cup coconut sugar
2 tablespoons honey
1 tablespoon ground cinnamon

1. Combine all ingredients in a glass jar and mix thoroughly.
2. Seal shut and use as needed in the shower.

24. CINNAMON-BASED FOUNDATION

Foundation is immensely helpful in helping smooth out skin, absorb grease, conceal blemishes, and reduce redness. Essentially, it creates an even canvas for the rest of your makeup, but it also works on its own to create a natural glow.

Foundation has been used throughout the centuries—but most of it was toxic. For example, in Ancient Greece and Rome—and even into the Middle Ages and the Elizabethan Age—foundation made with deadly white lead was used to make women's complexions fairer. Women who painted their faces with this mixture experienced side effects such as rotten teeth, hair loss, and even death.[16]

Over the years, the formula changed to become less toxic, but there was not a large variety of shades and the ingredients continued to be questionable. In the technicolor film era of Hollywood, powder foundation was introduced. It was meant to create a more natural look and was made out of dried and crushed pigments and oils. It was also during this time that liquid foundation was invented—for your legs.[17]

Nowadays, you can find liquid, powder, cream, and even stick foundations. Each type has its own benefits and provides a varying amount of coverage, but there are still challenges foundation-buyers face. Many common foundation brands still have toxins (less scary than lead, but still harmful) in their formulas, as well as common skin-clogging ingredients, like mineral oil. Not only that, but many brands do not have a wide-enough variety of shades for consumers to choose from and match to their natural skin tone.

Because your skin absorbs what you put on it, it's important you only put on the cleanest ingredients.[18] If you're looking to cover up any blemishes, oiliness, or redness but don't want to risk using a store-bought foundation, this DIY recipe is so clean, you can eat it if you want (though we don't recommend it—it doesn't taste great). The cacao powder provides color, while the cinnamon gives it depth and a blood-circulating effect.

HOMEMADE CINNAMON FOUNDATION POWDER

2 tablespoons zinc oxide or arrowroot powder

2 tablespoons arrowroot flour (you can find this in many baking stores or online)

2 teaspoons clay powder (optional, but I recommend bentonite clay, kaolin clay, or French green clay to help soak up oil)

2 tablespoons unsweetened 100% organic cacao powder (vary depending on your skin tone)

1/2 teaspoon organic ground cinnamon (vary depending on your skin tone)

1. Combine all ingredients except for the cacao powder and cinnamon.

2. Slowly add the cacao powder and cinnamon until the mixture closely matches your skin tone.
3. Shake well and store in an airtight container.
4. Apply using a large powder foundation brush.

25. TEETH WHITENER

Proper oral hygiene isn't just important for maintaining fresh breath; it's also important for preventing disease and improving your overall health. Poor dental health has been linked to various diseases, such as cardiovascular disease, stroke, diabetes, and dementia. One theory Dr. Peter Alldritt, Chairman of the Oral Health Committee at the Australian Dental Association, suggests is that "bacteria from your mouth can travel through the bloodstream and set up inflammation elsewhere in the blood vessels in the cardiovascular system."[19]

That's why it is vital to brush your teeth at least twice daily in order to maintain proper oral health. But *what* you brush your teeth with is also important. Most store-bought toothpaste contains sulphates, gums, artificial flavors, sweeteners, and binding agents created to help make toothpaste more palatable. Think about the amount of toothpaste you likely ingest while you're brushing your teeth—these ingredients are going directly into your body!

That's why dentist Thomas P. Connelly says, "I feel the more natural [with toothpaste] you can get, the better off you are." We can take a note from the Chinese, who first created a version of better-flavored toothpaste around 500 BCE by adding herbal products like ginseng, mint, and salt.[20]

This homemade toothpaste uses coconut oil, which has

antibacterial properties; baking soda, which can whiten teeth while being largely non-abrasive; and cinnamon essential oil, which has antifungal properties.[21]

CINNAMON WHITENING TOOTHPASTE

4 tablespoons organic coconut oil, melted
4 tablespoons baking soda
1 tablespoon xylitol powder or stevia (optional, can use less if needed)
15 drops cinnamon essential oil
10 drops peppermint essential oil
3 drops tea tree oil

1. Combine all ingredients and mix thoroughly.
2. Store in a glass jar in a cool location and use as needed.

26. DRY SHAMPOO

Whether you're avoiding over-shampooing your hair or just need a quick touch-up without a full wash, dry shampoo has your back. It's designed to soak up the oil in your hair, providing your hair with a quick refresh. It was first produced in the 1940s and was made out of fuller's earth, which is a clay that can soak up oil without harsh treatment (like bentonite clay).[22]

Since then, dry shampoo has gone through various forms; now there are spray (aerosol) and powder versions. Spray versions are primarily composed of alcohol plus cornstarch or clay, while powder versions are usually made of clay, talc, and starch, without the presence of alcohol.[23] The starch helps absorb the oil in your hair without over-drying it. When you add cinnamon essential oil to the mix (like in the recipe below), you get the additional benefits of stimulating blood circulation, which makes for a healthy scalp.

CINNAMON CACAO DRY SHAMPOO

1/4 cup cornstarch or arrowroot powder

2 tablespoons cacao powder (vary depending on your hair color)

4 drops cinnamon essential oil

1. Combine all ingredients together in a glass jar and shake vigorously. If you have dark hair, slowly add more cacao powder to obtain a color that resembles your hair color.

2. Use sparingly as needed on the roots of your hair. You can apply it with a powder brush or your fingers.

3. Let it set for 2–3 minutes before working it through with either your fingers or a brush.

27. BRONZER

Not only can bronzer give you a sun-kissed glow even in the dead of winter, but it can also come in handy if you are going to use contouring to shape your face. Contouring, or using makeup to define or minimize features on your face, was popularized by celebrities like the Kardashians, but it actually originated decades ago from within the drag community.[24]

To properly contour your face, you will need a product darker than your skin shade, which is where bronzer comes in. Bronzer should only be used for contouring when it's matte (like the DIY version below); shimmery bronzer draws light to areas, whereas contouring bronzer creates the illusion of shadows on your face.

Like many other cosmetics, bronzer comes in a few different forms: cream, gel, loose powder, and pressed powder. Typically, loose powder looks the most natural and is the easiest to blend. The powder bronzer recipe below uses natural ingredients;

unsweetened cacao powder gives the bronzer the dark color, while cinnamon and nutmeg give the bronzer more of a dimensional look.

CINNAMON COCOA BRONZER

1 tablespoon organic cornstarch or arrowroot powder
1 1/2 tablespoons organic unsweetened cacao powder (vary depending on your skin tone)
1 teaspoon (or less) organic cinnamon powder
1 teaspoon (or less) organic nutmeg

1. Place the cornstarch or arrowroot powder in a bowl.
2. Slowly add the cacao powder until it gets to your desired darkness. I recommend trying to match the color to one of your old bronzers or a sample from a makeup store.
3. Once you get your desired color, add tiny amounts of cinnamon and nutmeg to round out the color.
4. Store the bronzer in an old, cleaned-out mineral makeup jar or a clean glass jar.
5. Apply with a fluffy bronzer brush as desired.

HOW TO CONTOUR WITH BRONZER:

1. To define your cheekbones, suck your lips in to create a "fish face." You'll see hollows appear below your cheeks, forcing your cheekbones to look more prominent.
2. Place the bronzer in the hollows under your cheeks. Because the bronzer is darker than your natural skin tone, it will create the illusion of shadows below your cheekbones, making your cheeks look more defined and creating the look of a slimmer or more angular face.
3. You can also dust bronzer on your neck and on the sides of your face to create a slimming effect.

NUTRITION

BEAUTY

HEALTH

HOME

NUTRITION

BEAUTY

HEALTH

HOME

28. HELP TREAT ALOPECIA SYMPTOMS

Alopecia areata, also known as spot baldness, is an autoimmune disease where patches of hair are lost from the head, face, or other parts of the body. It's present in people of all ages, sexes, and ethnic groups and affects as many as 6.8 million people in the United States, according to the National Alopecia Areata Foundation.[25] It's a genetic disease, but *both* parents must have the genes to pass it on to their children (which is known as a "polygenic disease").

Some people may choose to shave their head and face so the bald spots are not apparent; others wear wigs or choose hairstyles to help cover up the bare spots. Unfortunately, there is no treatment that works for everyone with alopecia. Because it's an autoimmune disorder, it means your body's own immune system is attacking the hair follicles, causing hair to fall out. There are two routes for treatment: either suppress the immune system or stimulate hair growth; however, none of the current treatments or medications have been approved by the FDA (Food and Drug Administration).

While there are no holistic treatments that suppress the immune system, there *are* holistic treatments to help stimulate hair growth. Cinnamon leaf extract helps to enhance hair growth, which is why cinnamon essential oil has been found to possibly treat alopecia.[26] It's an easy, cheap, and low-risk way to help stimulate regrowth of your hair.

This hair and scalp mask not only helps boost circulation, but it also nourishes the hair that is already present on your head, thanks to the extra virgin olive oil, honey, and egg.

CINNAMON HAIR AND SCALP MASK

2 tablespoons extra virgin olive oil

2 drops cinnamon essential oil

1 tablespoon honey

1 egg

1. Crack the egg into a bowl and whisk.
2. Add the remaining ingredients and whisk to combine.
3. Apply the mask on your hair and scalp—I recommend massaging it into your scalp and working it all the way through to the ends.
4. Cover your hair with a shower cap or plastic bag and let the mask sit for 20–30 minutes.
5. Shampoo the mask out in the shower (it may take two shampoos) and condition as usual.

29. LIP-PLUMPING LIP BALM

Take a look at the success of brands like Kylie Cosmetics's lip kit and you'll get a taste of just how popular "bee-stung" lips are. Inspired by celebrities like Angelina Jolie, Kylie Jenner, and Scarlett Johansson, women have been searching for ways to create plumper, fuller lips for the past two decades. In fact, the American Society of Plastic Surgeons reported from 2000 to 2018, there was a 66 percent increase in lip augmentation procedures.[27]

There are a variety of ways to get fuller lips, ranging from fairly inexpensive (lip-plumping glosses) to expensive (lip injections). If you search the internet, you might also see teens resorting to dangerous methods (like using shot glasses) to create a puffi-er-looking pout, but those methods should *not* be replicated.

Cinnamon can help safely create the look of plumper lips. It contains cassia oil, which increases blood circulation.[28] Adding a little cinnamon essential oil to the lip balm recipe below helps boost circulation to your lips, making them look fuller. If you want an easy lip-plumping gloss, you can also take your favorite lip gloss and add 2–3 drops of cinnamon essential oil. Be sure to add them slowly and blend thoroughly so the cinnamon oil is evenly distributed.

CINNAMON LIP-PLUMPING BALM

1 tablespoon cocoa butter
1 tablespoon beeswax
1 tablespoon honey
1/2 tablespoon shea butter
1/2 tablespoon coconut oil
5 drops cinnamon essential oil

1. Combine all ingredients in a small, heat-safe bowl.
2. Create a double broiler by bringing a pot of water to boil, then placing the heat-safe bowl in the water (make sure no water goes in the bowl).
3. Mix thoroughly until melted.
4. Pour into a small glass jar and let cool.
5. Use as needed when your lips need moisture and/or some plumping action.

30. CELLULITE-FIGHTING BODY CREAM

If you've found cottage cheese–looking areas or dimples on your body, you're not alone. Those areas are caused by cellulite, and an estimated 80–98 percent of women will have cellulite at some point during their life.[29]

Cellulite is caused by the pressure of fat underneath the surface of your skin pulling against the fascia (web-like connective tissue) in your body. This creates the dimpled appearance you may see on the surface of your skin.

There's a common misconception that cellulite is synonymous with weight gain, but that's not always the case. In fact, people of all body types can have cellulite—even very thin people. Genetics play a huge factor in the presence and location of cellulite. For example, only an estimated 10 percent of men have cellulite.[30] This is because men's connective tissue is built differently than women's, making it harder for cellulite to appear.

There's no "cure" for cellulite, but there *are* ways to make it appear less visible. These treatments range from DIY home treatments, to creams and scrubs, to treatments done by professionals, such as light therapy, cool sculpting, and surgery.[31] In fact, the market for cellulite treatment is expected to exceed more than $2 billion by 2024, according to Market Watch.

That being said, there are some steps you can take to prevent additional cellulite from appearing without spending an arm and a leg. Having healthy skin is one of those steps; if your skin maintains its elasticity, the appearance of cellulite can be reduced. Maintaining healthy blood flow is another step to help prevent cellulite from forming. Because cinnamon helps boost blood circulation, the DIY body cream below not only helps you maintain moisturized and healthy skin, but also helps increase your circulation!

CITRUS CINNAMON CELLULITE-FIGHTING WHIPPED BODY CREAM

1 cup extra virgin coconut oil
5 drops orange essential oil
5 drops grapefruit essential oil
5 drops cinnamon essential oil

1. Place coconut oil in a large bowl. Using a hand whisk or an electric mixer, whisk thoroughly until the coconut oil is light and fluffy.
2. Add the essential oils and continue whisking until the oils have been evenly distributed.
3. Spoon into a glass jar and store in a cool, dark place until use.

31. ANTI-CELLULITE BODY SCRUB

Speaking of cellulite, you can create a whole anti-cellulite regime at home. While the routine won't cure cellulite, it can help reduce its appearance. It also helps you carve out some time for self-care.

Before using any body scrub in the shower, it is a good idea to first dry-brush your skin. This jump-starts your circulation and helps remove dead skin—something the Native Americans and Greeks have practiced for centuries.[32]

The cinnamon- and caffeine-based body scrub below helps exfoliate even further. Caffeine is popular in cellulite scrubs because of its ability to dehydrate your fat cells and make them look less visible.[33] Cinnamon helps boost circulation even further, plumping your skin and helping the cellulite look less apparent.

After you shower, dry off and use the cellulite-fighting cream on page "30. Cellulite-Fighting Body Cream" on page 73 to keep your newly exfoliated skin moisturized and firm.

CAFFEINE-BOOSTING ANTI-CELLULITE BODY SCRUB

1 cup coffee grounds (fresh or used, but used saves some money!)

1/2 cup extra virgin coconut oil

3 tablespoons coarse sugar (I recommend turbinado or coconut)

5 drops cinnamon essential oil

2 drops frankincense essential oil

1. Combine all ingredients in a large bowl.
2. Spoon into a clean glass jar and store in a cool, dry place until use.

32. ACNE-FIGHTING OIL CLEANSER

Have you tried cleanser after cleanser that promises to get rid of your acne, without any success? That's why there are so many acne-fighting cleansers on the market—it's hard to find a cleanser that works perfectly for you. Additionally, many cleansers contain harsh chemicals that can actually *trigger* acne, not fight it.

However, there is a cleanser you can make right from your own home that can help fight acne—an oil cleanser. If you've never tried oil cleansing, it can sound counterintuitive. After all, if acne is caused by excess oil production in our skin, why would you add more oil on top of it?[34]

The answer is a "like-dissolves-like" situation. When our skin is clogged by hardened oils that have settled into our pores (usually in the form of blackheads), plant-based oils can help dissolve these oils and clear our pores.

Many people who have acne tend to over-cleanse their skin out of fear that acne is caused by dirty skin. The problem with that? Washing your face too often strips your skin of its natural moisture, causing it to overproduce. And that results in—you guessed it—more clogged pores. Because oil is deeply hydrating, it can help your skin balance out and control oil production.

Not all oils are created equal, however. The comedogenic scale measures how likely skincare ingredients are to clog your pores. Some oils, like coconut oil, are high on this scale and can actually clog your skin even further. Other oils, like hemp seed oil, are low on the comedogenic scale and have a very low chance of clogging your pores.[35]

The DIY oil cleanser below uses a mix of low comedogenic oils as the base. It also has cinnamon essential oil and tea tree oil to help fight acne—both oils have known antibacterial properties.

ACNE-FIGHTING oil CLEANSER

1 ounce castor oil
2 ounces hemp seed oil
0.5 ounces argan oil
0.5 ounces jojoba oil

5 drops tea tree oil

3 drops neroli oil

3 drops cinnamon essential oil

1. Combine all oils in a glass bottle (preferably one with a dark tint) and shake to mix.

HOW TO OIL-CLEANSE USING THE DOUBLE-CLEANSING METHOD:

1. Take approximately 1–2 tablespoons of your oil cleanser and massage into your face.
2. Rinse off with warm water, then use your regular cleanser to cleanse again.
3. Follow with your regular skincare routine.

33. COZY BATH SALTS

Many people equate bath time to luxury—and for good reason. It can be incredibly relaxing to soak in a tub full of warm water (and maybe even bubbles). It's the epitome of self-care—it gives you time to read, nap, drink wine, do a face mask . . . maybe all of the above!

Baths can be more than just a de-stressing activity, though. Athletes, especially runners, have been using Epsom salt (magnesium sulfate) baths for years. By soaking in these natural minerals, you can get a variety of benefits. Epsom salt baths have been known to help in combating magnesium deficiency, fighting off colds, easing muscle aches, and improving sleep.[36]

Unfortunately, buying bath salts can be expensive, especially if you want to get fancy with scented baths. The good news? It's quite easy to make your own! The recipe below gives you a cozy, luxurious bath experience to help you de-stress and soak away any sore muscles.

COZY AND LUXURIOUS BATH SALTS

2 cups coarse sea salt

2 cups Epsom salt

2 tablespoons ground cinnamon

5 drops cinnamon essential oil

5 drops clove essential oil

5 drops vanilla essential oil

1 cup dried rose petals (optional)

1. Combine all ingredients together until evenly mixed.
2. Store in a glass jar.

HOW TO USE:

1. As your bathtub is filling with warm-hot water, add 2–3 tablespoons of the bath salts.
2. Get in, sit back, relax, and enjoy!

34. EXFOLIATING SOAP BARS

Soap is by no means a modern invention; the Ancient Babylonians were making soap as early as 2800 BCE. Their soap was made from fats mixed with ashes and was primarily used for cleaning wool before making it into cloth.[37] In 1550 BCE, the Ancient Egyptians had a similar notion—they mixed both animal and vegetable oils with alkaline salts to create their own soap.

Throughout the rest of history, various civilizations continued to make soap out of some form of oil, fat, and salt. Unlike our modern-day soaps, however, these soaps were used for cleaning the house or household items, like pots and pans, rather than the body.

These days, we have a variety of soaps as well: dish soap, hand soap, body soap, face soap . . . the list goes on and on. Although the formulation of gels has made soap bars a little less popular, they can be a travel-friendly personal hygiene item and even bring you a little luxury while on the road.

The recipe below combines cinnamon for blood circulation and oatmeal for exfoliation to create a sweet-smelling soap you can use for yourself or give as a gift.

CINNAMON OATMEAL EXFOLIATING SOAP BARS

4-8 ounce block of clear glycerin soap base (you can get this on Amazon)
2 tablespoons olive oil
2 tablespoons water
1/4 cup old-fashioned oats
1 tablespoon ground cinnamon

1. Cut the glycerin soap block into evenly sized cubes and melt them in the microwave in 30-second intervals. Stir between each interval to break up any clumps.
2. When all of the soap is melted, let it cool slightly. Then add the olive oil, water, oats, and cinnamon.
3. Stir ingredients together. Keep mixing for 1–3 minutes or until the mixture starts to thicken.
4. Pour the soap into a soap mold or repurposed empty container. Allow it to cool and harden (at least 1 hour).
5. Pop the soap out of the mold and store in a dry, cool place. Use within 3 months.

NUTRITION

BEAUTY

HEALTH

HOME

35. BATH BOMBS

Have you ever dropped an Alka-Seltzer tablet into a glass of water? Or any other dissolving tablet into a glass of liquid? If yes, then you know how bath bombs work.

The rainbow spheres were popularized in the 2010s for their ability to make bath time fun again. Once dropped into your bath, they dissolve and turn your bath into different colors and scents.

It works because the sodium bicarbonate (baking soda) in the bath bomb reacts with citric acid (or, in our recipe below, cream of tartar) to release carbon dioxide, making the bath bomb fizz and dissolve.[38]

For a bath bomb experience of your own, make some at home with the recipe below and plop one in your next bath! They also make great homemade gifts, especially if you use food coloring to make them various colors.

LUXURIOUS BATH BOMBS

1/2 teaspoon vanilla extract
1/4 teaspoon safflower oil
2 drops cinnamon essential oil
1/8 cup dried lavender
2 tablespoons baking soda
1 tablespoon cornstarch
1 tablespoon Epsom salt
1/2 tablespoon cream of tartar
Food coloring (optional; liquid is okay, but a dry/powdered food coloring is recommended)

1. Add the vanilla extract, safflower oil, and cinnamon essential oil to a small bowl and mix together. If you are using a liquid food coloring, combine it now with the liquid ingredients.
2. Combine the dry ingredients in a bowl. If you are using a dry/powdered food coloring, combine it with the dry ingredients.
3. Slowly pour the wet ingredients into the bowl of dry ingredients.
4. Whisk until the mixture has started to clump together.
5. Spoon the mixture into a silicone or plastic mold (you can use ice cube trays or mini muffin molds).
6. Use a spoon to pack the mixture down tightly.
7. Leave the bath bombs to dry for 10 hours before using.
8. If storing before use, allow the bath bombs to dry for at least 24 hours.

36. FOOT PEEL

We commonly do masks and peels for our face, but what about the rest of our body? Like our feet, for example. It's quite easy to take them for granted—after all, they're all the way at the bottom of our bodies, so we rarely see them up close.

But they do so much work for us! From carrying us around in our daily lives, to being squished into uncomfortable shoes, to being dried out on the beach in the summer, they go through a lot.

And because of that, they often show signs of wear. It's common for people to have cracked heels, calluses, and dry and rough skin on their feet. If the cracks are bad enough, they can deepen and become painful—maybe even infected.

To avoid this and keep your feet soft and healthy, you should exfoliate and use foot peels to slough off dead skin.[39] This can be done using a variety of methods. Chemical exfoliants tend to be the most effective—they serve to dissolve the dead skin, so you can slough the peeling skin off with a foot file or scrub. The home-made scrub below uses aspirin tablets to help exfoliate the skin and contains cinnamon oil to keep your skin bacteria-free. After exfoliating, make sure your feet are clean and moisturized—use a thick balm on your newly soft feet and wear natural socks to lock the moisture in.

SMᵒOTH-AS-BABY-FEET FOOT PEEL

1 capful of non-coated aspirin tablets (they should be white on the outside rather than the typical pink-red color of the coated tablets)

2 tablespoons lemon juice

2 tablespoons water

2 drops cinnamon essential oil

1. Pour aspirin tablets in a bowl and crush thoroughly.
2. Add the rest of the ingredients and mix well.
3. Apply the paste to the bottom of your feet, especially over any cracks.
4. Cover feet tightly with plastic wrap.
5. Put a thick pair of socks on over the plastic wrap and let sit for at least an hour.
6. Rinse your feet in warm water and pat dry, making sure to dry off any flakes of skin that have started shedding.
7. Apply a thick moisturizing balm (like Aquaphor) or coconut oil to your feet before putting on a clean pair of thick socks to help lock in the moisture.
8. It's normal for skin to continue shedding over the next few days. Continue to keep your feet moisturized!

37. REDUCE FINE LINES

Did you know that after age twenty-five, you start losing collagen and there is no way to prevent it? But don't worry—there *are* things you can do to increase collagen production in your body.

But first, let's backtrack. What *is* collagen and why is it important?

Collagen is a protein your body naturally produces; it's found in many essential parts of your body, like your bones, muscles, skin, teeth, and nails.[40] It is derived from the Greek word *kolla*, meaning "glue," which is appropriate—you can think of collagen as the "glue" that binds your body together.

Cinnamon promotes collagen I biosynthesis in dermal fibroblasts, which are the cells in the layer of your skin called the dermis.[41] These cells are important for generating connective tissue and helping repair your skin from any injury. Collagen also helps with skin elasticity, which gives you a youthful glow because elastic skin will not sag or wrinkle as easily as non elastic skin.

Consuming cinnamon and collagen supplements can help you boost collagen production, creating an anti-aging effect.[42]

38. GET A SUNLESS GLOW

Want a healthy-looking tan without hitting the beach or the tanning salon? Understandable, seeing as spending too much time soaking up the sun's rays or the tanning salon's light can have harmful consequences. At the very least, the UV (ultraviolet) rays from the sun or artificial tanning device can cause sunburn, but did you know the "tan" color your skin turns is a result of DNA damage? Too much UV exposure can also lead to chemical hypersensitivity, speed up aging, and even result in carcinoma (skin cancer).[43]

That's where DIY bronzing lotion comes in. It helps you achieve a tan glow without the sun or a tanning bed. It uses cocoa powder and cinnamon to create a bronze color while moisturizing your skin at the same time.

SUNLESS BRONZING LOTION

1/3 cup 100% cocoa powder (vary depending on your skin tone)
1 tablespoon cornstarch or arrowroot powder
1 teaspoon cinnamon
1 teaspoon mica powder (optional, for shimmer)
8 ounces plain body lotion

1. Combine the cocoa powder, cornstarch/arrowroot powder, and cinnamon in a small bowl; mix well.

2. If you desire a deeper color, continue adding cocoa powder until you achieve the color you want.

3. If you desire a shimmery bronzing lotion, add the mica powder.

4. Mix thoroughly into your body lotion (you may have to use a whisk to ensure it is mixed evenly).

5. Apply as needed.

CHAPTER 3

FOR THE HEALTH ENTHUSIAST IN YOU

NUTRITION

BEAUTY

HEALTH

HOME

39. MAKE THROAT LOZENGES

Suffering from a cold? Cinnamon is one of the most powerful spices to help you recover from the common cold. It's a great source of antioxidants and has several healing properties, including antinociceptive effects (meaning it helps block the sensation of pain).[1] The cinnamon in this homemade throat lozenge recipe helps alleviate the pain of a sore throat, and the other natural ingredients make these lozenges healthier for you than commercial lozenges.

Typical throat lozenges contain a large amount of sugar and processed ingredients, which can actually make you feel worse as your body tries to heal. Furthermore, most store-bought throat lozenges contain compounds that cause drowsiness, which makes going about your everyday life difficult. Also, the active compounds amylmetacresol and dichlorobenzyl alcohol (which are components of most over-the-counter throat lozenges) have been proven to be noneffective antivirals.[2]

These homemade throat lozenges use natural ingredients to soothe your throat and fight bacteria: manuka honey has significant antibacterial effects,[3] cinnamon has antibacterial properties,[4] ginger and sage help boost your immune system,[5] and eucalyptus oil provides a cooling effect (similar to menthol in store-bought lozenges).

CINNAMON HONEY THROAT LOZENGES

1/2 knob whole fresh ginger, peeled and chopped into large segments
1 cinnamon stick
1 bunch fresh sage
1 cup water
1 lemon
1/2 cup manuka honey
1/2 cup raw sugar
2-4 drops eucalyptus essential oil (optional)

1. Place the ginger, cinnamon, sage, and water in a medium saucepan. Bring to a boil over high heat, then cover with a lid and simmer on low heat for 10–15 minutes.

2. While the water is simmering, zest the lemon. Then cut the lemon in half and squeeze the juice into a small bowl.

3. Remove the ginger, cinnamon, and sage from the water. Add the honey, sugar, lemon juice, and lemon zest to the water and stir until the honey and sugar are dissolved. Turn the heat up to high so the mixture comes to a boil again.

4. Closely monitor the saucepan for signs the mixture is ready: the water will start to evaporate and the mixture will change to a golden caramel color. Alternatively, you can use a candy thermometer; the mixture is ready when the temperature reaches 300°F.

5. Carefully pour the liquid into a silicone mold. Cool at room temperature for at least 2 hours.

6. Remove from the mold. Cut wax paper or beeswax wraps into 6 x 6-inch squares and place the cough drop inside, then wrap tightly. If desired, you can then wrap these in aluminum foil to make sure the drops stay enclosed.

7. Store in a cool dark location and enjoy as needed!

NUTRITION

BEAUTY

HEALTH

HOME

40. MAKE HOMEMADE COUGH SYRUP

A common symptom of winter colds is a persistent cough. Whether you're seeking relief for the dry cough or just want something to soothe your inflamed throat, cough syrup is probably your go-to remedy. Over-the-counter cough syrups and suppressants can make you drowsy, and many contain dextromethorphan (DXM), which can cause psychedelic effects if taken at too high of a dosage.[6] This homemade blend, on the other hand, has all natural ingredients to ease your cough without making you feel sleepy or dosing yourself with chemicals.

Raw honey helps soothe your throat because of its antibacterial, antimicrobial, and anti-inflammatory properties.[7] Apple cider vinegar, lemon, and cayenne can help clear mucus out of your throat (which helps you get rid of that phlegmy cough), while cinnamon is an antimicrobial that will help kill the cold germs that caused the cough in the first place!

CINNAMON APPLE CIDER VINEGAR COUGH SYRUP

4 cups water
1 cup raw, local honey
1/4 cup lemon juice (fresh or bottled)
2 tablespoons apple cider vinegar
1 tablespoon cinnamon powder
1 teaspoon cayenne pepper
1/4 knob ginger, grated (or 3 tablespoons ginger powder, but fresh is better)

1. Boil the water then lower to a simmer.
2. Add all ingredients and simmer until the volume is reduced by half.
3. Strain using a cheesecloth or a fine mesh strainer.
4. Store in a glass jar in the fridge and use 1–2 spoonfuls as needed. Can be stored for up to 2 months.

....

41. CREATE YOUR OWN MOuTHWASH

Floss, brush, rinse, mouthwash—this is how the typical oral hygiene routine goes. Mouthwash—the last step—is important because it not only helps freshen your breath, but can also help prevent plaque, gingivitis, and tooth decay.[8] If your gums are bleeding after you floss, mouthwash can be even more vital because it will help sanitize your mouth.

Typical store-bought mouthwashes cost at least $5, so you'll save big bucks over time by using a homemade mouthwash. Thanks to its cinnamon and tea tree oil (natural antibacterials) and baking soda (the base of many natural mouthwashes), this inexpensive, homemade mouthwash tastes great *and* helps prevent bacterial overgrowth, re-mineralize enamel, and reduce cavities.[9]

CLEANSING CINNAMON MOuTHWASH
2 cups distilled water (or boiled and cooled water)
1 tablespoon baking soda
1 teaspoon sea salt
2 drops of cinnamon essential oil
1 drop tea tree oil

NUTRITION

BEAUTY

HEALTH

HOME

1. Mix all ingredients well in a mason jar.
2. Shake vigorously before using 1 tablespoon as needed.

42. MAKE AN OIL-PULLING BLEND

This ancient practice helps reduce plaque, gingivitis, bad breath, and fungus in your mouth. According to ancient Indian Ayurvedic text, oil pulling can be used for the prevention and treatment of more than thirty different illnesses, from mild ailments—such as headaches, migraines, thrombosis, and eczema—to fatal diseases—such as diabetes and asthma.[10] The fatty acids of the oil bind to any fungus in your mouth, so after you spit it out, it's gone!

Oil pulling has become more common in the past few years due to the rising popularity of Ayurvedic practices and holistic health. Many holistic brands now sell their own oil-pulling blends, which are made of various essential oils and carrier oils, but you can easily make your own for a fraction of the price. This homemade blend uses coconut oil for its extra antibacterial properties, plus cinnamon essential oil, which is a natural antifungal. With regular use, this blend helps prevent fungus.

HOMEMADE OIL-PULLING BLEND

1 cup extra virgin coconut oil
1/2 cup extra virgin olive oil or sesame oil
4 drops cinnamon essential oil

1. Melt the coconut oil in a pot or the microwave.
2. Remove from the heat and add the olive/sesame oil and cinnamon essential oil.

3. Whisk with a fork and store in a glass jar.

HOW TO USE:

1. Vigorously swish 1–2 teaspoons of oil in your mouth each morning.
2. Continue for 5 to 20 minutes.
3. Spit out and follow by brushing your teeth, flossing, and using mouthwash.

....

43. TREAT ATHLETE'S FOOT

An estimated 3–15 percent of people in the United States, at some point in their life, will get athlete's foot—a common fungal infection that occurs when your feet come into contact with fungus in warm, moist areas.[11] It usually develops between your toes and can be caused by anything from sweaty feet in an unaerated shoe or sock, to bare feet with cuts in a locker room. If you have allergies, eczema, a genetic predisposition, a weakened immune system, naturally sweaty feet, or circulation problems, you may be more prone to contracting athlete's foot at some point in your life.

Athlete's foot is most commonly presented in the space between your littlest toe and the toe beside it; symptoms include flaky skin in the affected area, reddened and cracked skin, and swelling. While it's not usually dangerous, it can be *quite* annoying. Luckily, you can treat it at home!

An easy solution (that also feels like a spa treatment!) is a relaxing cinnamon foot soak. Cinnamon, tea tree oil, and white

NUTRITION

BEAUTY

HEALTH

HOME

NUTRITION

vinegar—proven antifungals—create a home remedy that will help cure athlete's foot over time.

RELAXING FOOT SOAK

4 cinnamon sticks (or you can use 2 drops of cinnamon essential oil)
2 drops tea tree oil
1/2 cup white vinegar

1. Fill a large bowl (big enough to fit both your feet) with boiled water that has been allowed to cool to a temperature you can comfortably soak your feet in.
2. Add all the ingredients.
3. Soak for up to an hour and dry your feet thoroughly. Repeat each night until the athlete's foot disappears.

BEAUTY

44. BOOST YOUR MEMORY

My mom always told me to eat cinnamon and honey before a test (usually in the form of cinnamon honey peanut butter toast) to boost my memory. Turns out, there's actually some science behind this . . .

Cinnamon is a powerful brain booster—it contains phytochemicals that boost your brain's ability to burn glucose and function. Studies show that with consumption of glucose, people find positive effects on both long- and short-term memory, as well as cognitive performance.[12]

The compounds in cinnamon that give it its flavor and aroma are "metabolized into sodium benzoate in the liver. Sodium benzoate then becomes the active compound, which readily enters the brain and stimulates hippocampal plasticity."[13] Simply put, cinnamon can help with memory aid and improve learning.

HEALTH

HOME

You can take a teaspoon of cinnamon mixed with wild, raw honey before a big exam, before studying, or every day as a memory supplement.

45. TREAT INSECT BITES

If you've ever had an unbelievably itchy insect bite, you know how annoying it can be. Insect bites itch because the insect's saliva triggers your body's histamine response (the same response you get when you're allergic to something). Your body's immune system then kicks into overdrive, increasing blood flow and increasing white blood cell count (your body's immune system defenders) around the area of the bite, causing inflammation, swelling, and that familiar itching feeling.

Even though the bite feels itchy, try to avoid scratching as much as possible. When you scratch, you're likely to break the skin and infect the bite with bacteria from your hands or your environment.

Luckily, cinnamon's antibacterial properties will help you ward off infection from the bite if you *do* scratch. Its anti-inflammatory properties can help the swelling subside as well. Both cinnamon and honey (a common superstar pairing) have powerful antibacterial properties and help your body heal.[14] Aloe vera, a common sunburn remedy, is known to help soothe your skin not only from burns, but from bites as well. Finally, camphor oil (a relative of cinnamon) helps soothe the itch even more and relax the muscles around the bite.

NUTRITION

ANTI-ITCH INSECT BITE PASTE

1 teaspoon ground cinnamon

1 teaspoon raw honey

1 teaspoon aloe vera gel (or 1 teaspoon fresh aloe vera flesh)

1 drop camphor oil (optional)

1. Mix all the ingredients together to form a thick paste.
2. Apply it on your bite and leave it for an hour.
3. To avoid attracting insects with the sweet honey, be sure to wash off the paste before going outside.

BEAUTY

46. MAKE SUPER-HEALING CHICKEN SOUP

Chicken noodle soup is a popular cold remedy. The broth helps you stay hydrated (loss of fluids can slow down healing when you're sick), while the chicken itself provides an easily digestible form of protein to support your immune system and act as a building block for your bones, muscles, skin, and blood.[15]

This ancient Chinese recipe takes regular chicken soup to another level with its additional healing properties. It combines herbs commonly used in traditional Chinese medicine with homemade bone broth. It's easier than you think—homemade broth is simply made by boiling the chicken! These ingredients work to combat cold symptoms and help your body heal faster.

HEALTH

HEALING CHINESE BLACK CHICKEN SOUP

6 dried shiitake mushrooms

4 pieces astragalus root (Huáng Qí (黄芪)), thinly sliced

3 pieces Angelica sinensis (Dāng Guī (当归)), thinly sliced

HOME

1 sweet potato or Chinese wild yam (Huái Shān (淮山))
1/2 knob ginger
1 black chicken (I recommend Silkie chicken (乌鸡), but any regular chicken works too)
6 cups water
1/4 cup dried goji berries
1/3 cup dried jujubes
1 cinnamon stick

1. Soak the mushrooms, astragalus root, and Angelica sinensis in a bowl of water for 30 minutes and then drain.
2. While those ingredients are soaking, chop the sweet potato into rounds and the ginger into thin slices.
3. Add the water and chicken to a large pot. Bring to a boil.
4. Add all ingredients to the boiling water and lower to a simmer.
5. Simmer for 30–40 minutes, or until the dried jujubes are soft and the chicken is soft enough to fall off the bone.
6. Season with salt and enjoy.

47. TREAT YEAST INFECTIONS AND BACTERIAL VAGINOSIS

Up to 75 percent of American women contract a vaginal yeast infection at least once in their lives. Another infection that has similar symptoms, but a different cause, is bacterial vaginosis (BV). BV is the most common vaginal infection among women aged fifteen to forty-four years and is often caused by an imbalance of good bacteria in the body.[16] In many of these cases, these women have recurring infections or symptoms.

It can be expensive to repeatedly buy over-the-counter medications or go to the doctor for antibiotics. Not to mention it's slightly embarrassing and quite annoying to take the time out of your day to schedule doctor's appointments. While these problems might go away on their own, the symptoms (itching, discharge, odor) make life unpleasant.

This recipe uses natural ingredients to help treat symptoms and, in some cases, the actual issue of yeast infections and bacterial vaginosis. This works because of cinnamon's natural antifungal properties, and tea tree oil and coconut oil both have antibacterial properties to help fight any imbalances. These ingredients can help reduce symptoms of yeast infections and bacterial infections, and even treat weak yeast infections or instances of BV.

HEALING CINNAMON SALVE

1 teaspoon cinnamon
2 drops tea tree oil
1 tablespoon coconut oil, melted

TO USE AS A SUPPOSITORY:

1. Mix all ingredients together.
2. Place an empty cardboard tampon applicator on a plate.
3. Fill with the cinnamon, tea tree oil, and coconut oil mixture.
4. Place in the freezer for 3 hours or until solidified. Insert as you would a tampon.
5. Allow the healing salve to melt completely and soothe the infected area.

TO USE TOPICALLY:

1. Mix ingredients together and use your fingers to spread all over the infected area.

Note: With both remedies, I recommend wearing a panty liner (to avoid oil stains) and using at night.

48. PREVENT CANDIDA OVERGROWTH

An estimated 1.4 million patient visits for vaginal candidiasis occur annually in the United States.[17] Candida is a fungus that's naturally produced by the body (men included!). This form of yeast serves to aid with digestion, but the issue arises when it begins to grow out of control. When that happens, it breaks down the intestine walls and penetrates the bloodstream.

Common symptoms of candida overgrowth are frequent yeast infections, skin or nail fungal infections (like athlete's foot), chronic fatigue, digestive issues (constipation, bloating, diarrhea), brain fog, carb and sugar cravings, and mood swings. In order to get candida back under control, there are a couple of steps holistic practitioners recommend taking:

First, starve the candida by removing or limiting refined sugars, alcohol, natural sugars (including honey and fruit), caffeine, and carbohydrates (including starchy veggies like sweet potatoes, grains, gluten, and legumes)—even though you may feel an intense craving for them.

Second, focus on high-fat and high-protein foods (similar to the keto diet) and help out the good bacteria in your gut by eating fermented foods, like sauerkraut and yogurt. Stick with this diet for two weeks.

Third, begin to consume antifungal foods. This is where cinnamon comes in.

Cinnamon is especially helpful when you're limiting your sugar intake because it helps food taste sweet without adding any sugar, thus curbing your sugar cravings. The even-better news? Cinnamon is an antifungal, which helps kill the candida overgrowth!

CINNAMON TEA

1 cinnamon stick
2 pieces fresh ginger
1 cup boiling water
1 drop oregano oil

1. Steep the cinnamon and ginger in the boiling water for 10 minutes.
2. Remove the cinnamon and ginger from the cup and add the oregano oil. Stir well.
3. Enjoy one to two cups per day.

CINNAMON KEFIR

1 cup unsweetened kefir
1 teaspoon cinnamon powder
1 teaspoon turmeric powder
1 teaspoon ground ginger
1 pinch black pepper

1. Whisk or blend all ingredients together and enjoy right away.

49. HELP SOoTHE MENSTRUAL CRAMPS

Is it that time of the month? If you're experiencing period cramps, know that you're not alone. Many women feel them before, during, and after their period—a condition known as dysmenorrhea. Because your uterine lining contracts and sheds during menstruation, it can result in a cramping sensation as a side effect. The intensity of your cramps can be determined by the levels of prostaglandins (a hormone-like substance) in your body—the higher the levels, the more pain you're likely to experience.

If you are older or have given birth, you are less likely to have severe cramps. On the other hand, if you have endometriosis, the lining that's typically inside your uterus forms *outside* it, resulting in a higher frequency and intensity of cramps.

Soothe any cramps you might have by making a warming cinnamon salve that you can massage on your stomach. It also works great to comfort a sore lower back or loosen up tight shoulders. Alternatively, to warm you from the inside out and help alleviate cramps, you can drink the alternate cinnamon tea recipe below.

WARMING CiNNAMoN SALVE

2 ounces beeswax
1/2 cup coconut oil
1/4 cup olive oil
3 tablespoons jojoba oil
1 tablespoon vitamin E oil
10 milliliters of 500mg CBD oil (optional)

10 drops cinnamon essential oil

8 drops sandalwood essential oil

4 drops clary sage essential oil

3 drops eucalyptus essential oil

1. Fill the bottom half of a double boiler halfway with water and place over medium to high heat.

2. Add the beeswax to the top of the double boiler. When the water starts to boil and the wax starts to melt, turn the heat down to low.

3. Stir occasionally to break up the wax.

4. Once the beeswax is melted, add the coconut oil, olive oil, jojoba oil, vitamin E oil, and CBD oil (if using); stir until combined and clear.

5. Add the essential oils and mix thoroughly again.

6. Pour the salve into a shallow container—I recommend you use glass, ceramic, or high-grade stainless steel—and let sit at room temperature until hardened.

7. Use on your low back and abdomen whenever needed! It should melt in your fingers as you apply.

CRAMP-SOOTHING CINNAMON TEA

2 cinnamon sticks

12 ounces water

1 tablespoon raw honey

1. Boil the cinnamon with the water.

2. Add the honey; stir until dissolved.

3. Enjoy two to three times per day.

50. HELP PREVENT CANCER

Cancer is a disease the world has been continuously fighting to prevent, yet there were still an estimated 18 million cases reported worldwide in 2018. The United States had the fifth highest cancer rate in the world that year, with 352 cases per one hundred thousand people.[18]

While there is no "cure" for cancer, there are multiple treatments that have proven effective. However, the best treatment is *prevention.*

There have been multiple studies on the suggestion that cinnamon extract may suppress tumor progression. This is because cinnamon can increase the activity of cancer-fighting cells (CD8(+) T cells). This is the same effect chemotherapy has—the killing of cancer cells. The researchers concluded "cinnamon extract has the potential to be an alternative medicine for tumor treatment."[19]

While cinnamon should not be a replacement for any medication, it can support your health if you take it regularly. It's quite easy (and delicious!) to add to your diet—think of sprinkling some on your coffee, oatmeal, or yogurt in the morning.

51. EASE TOoTHACHES

Have tooth pain? You're not alone. Toothaches are the most common cause of oral pain.[20] The pain can range from a sharp and stabbing feeling to a dull ache whenever pressure is applied to the affected spot. They can be caused by a variety of factors, including infection, cavities, tooth decay and fractures, and repetitive eroding motions, like chewing or teeth grinding.[21]

You can help prevent toothaches by practicing proper oral hygiene (like regularly brushing, flossing, and wearing a nightguard if you grind your teeth), but if you already have a toothache, don't worry—there are steps you can take to relieve your pain.

If bacteria or infection is the source of your pain, cinnamon can help. Cinnamon is known to have antimicrobial, antifungal, and anti-inflammatory effects.[22] This means it can help reduce localized swelling and fight the bacteria that's causing the ache. You can create a paste of cinnamon and honey to soothe your toothache, but if the pain persists, we recommend you visit your dentist to find a solution.

TOOTHACHE EASING BALM

5 teaspoons honey

1 teaspoon ground cinnamon

1. Mix the honey and cinnamon together thoroughly.
2. Apply to the affected area using a clean fingertip or cotton swab.

52. AID DIGESTION

There's nothing more dissatisfying than eating a great meal only to have an upset stomach afterward. Instead of reaching for over-the-counter medicines to find relief, try sipping on a cup of cinnamon tea. That's because cinnamon (even in small doses) helps lower your stomach's carbon dioxide levels, which aids with digestion.[23]

Incorporating cinnamon into your daily diet can help maintain proper digestive health; try sprinkling some on top of your food (see the recipe section of this book for more cinnamon recipes!).

Fun fact: It's not a new concept—ancestors as far back as first-century Romans used cinnamon as a remedy for many digestive ailments.[24]

DIGESTION-SOOTHING CINNAMON TEA

2 slices fresh ginger root
1 chamomile tea bag (or 1 tablespoon dried chamomile flowers)
1 cinnamon stick
1 cup boiling water
1 tablespoon raw honey

1. Place the ginger, chamomile, and cinnamon stick in a cup.
2. Pour boiling water over it and steep for 5–10 minutes.
3. Pour through a strainer and into another cup.
4. Stir in the honey and enjoy!

53. AVOID GAS

Passing gas is very human, but that doesn't stop it from being embarrassing. It can also feel physically uncomfortable—it often goes hand in hand with bloating.

The process starts when you swallow too much air or eat certain foods. The air or food moves down into your large intestine, where the bacteria in your body begin to break down these products, creating gas.

If you have digestion issues—like irritable bowel syndrome (IBS) and small intestinal bacterial overgrowth (SIBO)—or food intolerances and allergies—like lactose intolerance and Celiac's disease—you may be prone to gas.

Cinnamon is your secret weapon to avoiding this. It prevents the formation of gas by lowering your body's amount of stomach acid and pepsin (the main digestive enzyme in your stomach that breaks down proteins).[25]

In a recent gut-health study, researchers at the Melbourne, Australia–based RMIT University School of Engineering determined that even a small dose of cinnamon helps drop carbon dioxide levels in the stomach, which can lower body temperatures and aid digestion.

So sip on some cinnamon tea or incorporate cinnamon into your meals to ease your digestion and help prevent passing gas.

54. GET RID OF BAD BREATH

Bad breath, also known as halitosis, is caused by bacteria in the mouth. It's a common occurrence—about 30 percent of the world's population experiences some type of bad breath.[26] Most bad breath is temporary, meaning it occurs after eating certain foods, smoking tobacco, or not brushing the teeth.

However, if you have persistent bad breath, it could be signs of an underlying problem, including gum disease, dry mouth, poor oral hygiene, or a combination of these things. In small cases, more significant diseases like advanced liver or kidney disease may lead to bad breath as well. If you're experiencing severe symptoms (such as nausea and vomiting, shortness of breath, and/or fatigue) in addition to bad breath, it's recommended you visit your primary care physician.[27]

Because cinnamon has antibacterial properties, it helps kill the bacteria in your mouth that contribute to bad breath. To cure basic bad breath, you can use cinnamon in mouthwash form, toothpaste form, gum form, or simply sprinkling cinnamon in your water and drinking it.

55. HEAL WOuNDS

What's in your at-home first aid kit? Did you know you can clean and heal wounds with products right from your own kitchen?

Cinnamon is one of these "home-pantry first aid kit" products; the spice has been shown to improve wound healing.[28] The American Chemical Society has also reported the development of a new drug that uses cinnamon and peppermint oil to treat and heal chronic wounds and is effective against four different types of bacteria.[29] This is because cinnamaldehyde, the compound that gives cinnamon its distinctive taste and color, has antimicrobial properties.[30]

Honey is another powerful bacteria-killer, making it an ideal partner with cinnamon for wound healing. When properly used, honey can help clear infections and reduce the likelihood of scarring.

While you may be tempted to grab any honey off the shelf in times of emergency, manuka honey is recommended; it was approved by the US Federal Drug Administration in 2007 as an option for wound treatment.[31]

NUTRITION

BEAUTY

HEALTH

HOME

To help heal your wounds, mix 1 tablespoon manuka honey with 1 teaspoon of cinnamon powder (or 1 drop of cinnamon essential oil). If this is not enough to cover the wound, double the recipe. Apply the paste to the wound. Then take a typical wound dressing, like a gauze bandage roll, and wrap it tightly around the wound. Leave it on for 24 hours and change as needed.

56. HELP PROTECT YOUR GUT

Health starts from the inside out. While there has long been a focus on physical health, only recently has gut health stepped into the spotlight.

Gut health is important because of the gut–brain connection. Our GI (gastrointestinal) tract houses trillions of microorganisms. This is your gut microbiome and it influences your mood, health, appetite, and more.[32]

Contrary to popular belief, not all bacteria are bad. There are "good" bacteria in your gut, which is what probiotics and prebiotics help to support. But because everyone has a different gut microbiome, it's hard to determine which (and even if) commercial probiotics are effective. Prebiotics, on the other hand, help feed the healthy bacteria in your gut and are effective for most microbiomes.

It's important to provide your gut with adequate prebiotics because they're essentially the food that help the good bacteria thrive. Common prebiotics are resistant starches (like green bananas), dandelion greens, oats, and apples.

A lesser-known one? Cinnamon. It's known to have prebiotic properties that are helpful to the growth of good bacteria and can help suppress pathogenic bacteria.[33] Take a look at the recipe section for delicious ways to incorporate cinnamon in your diet!

57. HELP TREAT ECZEMA

Eczema is a skin condition that affects over 30 million Americans.[34] The word is derived from "to boil over" in Ancient Greek, which is a fitting indicator of the itchy, inflamed patches present on the skin when an eczema flare-up occurs. The patches of skin are usually dry and sensitive and can even swell or ooze.

There is no single known cause of eczema, but people who have eczema tend to have an over-reactive immune system. When the immune system is triggered by a certain substance, it reacts by creating inflammation in the body, resulting in the eczema patches. People's eczema triggers can vary, but common ones are stress, dry skin, infections, environmental allergens, hormones, and certain fragrances.[35]

Although there is no cure for eczema, there are a variety of treatments, ranging from topical over-the-counter drugs to home remedies, phototherapy, and more. The National Eczema Foundation recommends knowing and recognizing your personal eczema triggers, maintaining a proper bathing and moisturizing ritual, and using treatments as necessary to help manage your eczema flare-ups.

While consuming too much cinnamon may trigger eczema, it can be applied topically to help bring relief to dry eczema patches.[36] By creating the below paste and applying it to the affected area, you can moisturize the patch, relieve swelling and inflammation, and help prevent the patch from getting infected.

ECZEMA RELIEF PASTE

2 tablespoons honey
2 tablespoons cinnamon

1. Mix the honey and cinnamon together.
2. Apply liberally to the affected area; leave on for 20 minutes.
3. Wash off with warm water before moisturizing the area.

58. BOOST HEART HEALTH

Cardiovascular disease is a serious matter. The number one cause of death in the United States—across both genders and most races—is heart disease. It also costs a lot of money: Accounting for loss in worker productivity, medical bills, and medicine, the United States lost $219 billion from 2014 to 2015 due to heart disease complications.[37]

There are several risk factors for heart disease, including having diabetes, being overweight or obese, eating an unhealthy diet, using alcohol excessively, and not exercising enough. The three biggest factors, however, are smoking, high blood pressure, and high cholesterol levels.

Fortunately, we can mitigate risk by minimizing these risk factors. By slowly making lifestyle changes—like quitting smoking, eating a whole-food diet, moderating alcohol use, and exercising regularly—you can lower your risk for heart disease. High cholesterol levels are harder to tackle, but you can also manage that with your diet. This is because cholesterol comes from two sources:

1. **Your liver**, which makes all the cholesterol your body needs.
2. **Animal products you eat**, like meat and full-fat dairy products.

When you eat foods that are too high in trans fats and saturated fats, your liver starts to make more cholesterol than it needs, which increases your cholesterol level. However, not all cholesterol is bad. Cholesterol can be divided into two types:

1. **LDL cholesterol:** The "bad" cholesterol. It contributes to fat buildup in your arteries.
2. **HDL cholesterol:** The "good" cholesterol. It carries LDL cholesterol away from your arteries and back into your liver, thus preventing too much fatty build up.

It's important to have a balance of the two—too much bad cholesterol and your arteries can become clogged; too much good cholesterol can cause heart issues.[38]

Certain foods can help balance your cholesterol. Dark leafy greens, berries, and dark chocolate can all help lower your LDL cholesterol.[39] Cinnamon is an important food that can help *lower* your LDL cholesterol and *boost* your HDL cholesterol.[40] Recent studies have found that a daily dose of cinnamon is helpful for impacting your cholesterol levels, so now's the perfect time to start adding a pinch of cinnamon to your coffee, tea, yogurt, smoothies . . . the possibilities are endless!

59. REGULATE BLOOD SUGAR

Every year, 1.5 million Americans are diagnosed with diabetes. In 2018, over 10 percent of the United States population had diabetes.

This disease is quite prevalent and can be severe—it was reported as the seventh leading cause of death in the US in 2017, although the American Diabetes Association suspects the amount of diabetes-related deaths is underreported.[41]

To best understand diabetes, let's first look at what blood sugar is. Sugars from the food you eat turn into glucose in your bloodstream. Your body then uses insulin to help pull the glucose out of your bloodstream and into your cells. Having diabetes means something in this process is broken.

There are two types of diabetes:

1. **Type I:** This affects people of all ages, races, and sizes. People who have type I diabetes cannot *produce* enough insulin.
2. **Type II:** This is the most common form of diabetes. Although your body can properly produce insulin, if you have type II diabetes, your body cannot properly *use* its insulin.

There are also people who are pre-diabetic—people who are at risk of developing type II diabetes because of their higher-than-average blood sugar levels, but who don't have high enough blood sugar levels for it to be considered type II diabetes yet.

You can manage both forms of diabetes through exercise and a proper diet, although people with type I diabetes will typically need insulin treatments and injections. An important part of managing type II diabetes is controlling your blood glucose levels.

That's where cinnamon comes in! A 2003 study by the American Diabetes Association shows that diabetics who took cinnamon had lower glucose levels after forty days when compared to the placebo group.[42] A meta-analysis of ten studies in 2013 also showed a statistically significant decrease in blood glucose levels after taking cinnamon.[43]

Although cinnamon shouldn't be seen as a replacement for any medication, it can be a helpful supplement to help you naturally lower and control your blood sugar levels. By consuming it daily—especially in replacement of sugar—it can help control glucose levels for type II diabetics.

60. ENHANCE YOUR MOOD

Feeling depressed, anxious, or simply just down? Cinnamon can help boost your mood! It's been shown to have antidepressant effects in rats receiving lead acetate, but more than that, its effects on your blood sugar can explain why it has such a powerful effect on your mood.[44]

In recent years, there has been an increase in the number of studies linking blood sugar levels and mood disorders, such as depression. Because your brain runs largely on glucose, spikes or large dips in glucose levels can impact not only how your brain functions, but also your mood. To illustrate this relationship: About 25 percent of people with diabetes also suffer from depression.[45] Because cinnamon can help regulate your blood sugar, consuming it regularly can help you achieve more balanced moods.[46]

Another link to your mood is your gut's health. If you consume too much processed sugar or other gut-irritants, your mood can take a hit as well. That's because 90 percent of your serotonin receptors are located in your gut. Because serotonin, also known as the "happy chemical," is an important contributor to your happiness and well-being, it's vital these receptors work properly. To help cut down on the amount of sugar you consume, Harvard Medical

School's blog recommends you add cinnamon to your breakfast in place of sugar or sugar substitutes.[47]

61. STIMULATE LIBIDO

Cinnamon has been suggested as a treatment for sexual dysfunction in Ayurvedic medicine. A 2013 study looked into the validity of that statement by measuring sperm count and smooth muscle tissue in aged rats both before and after giving them cassia cinnamon for twenty-eight days. The study found there was an increase in sexual function, although sperm counts were unchanged. Therefore, the study concluded that while cinnamon does not help with male fertility (sperm count), it does aid in increasing sexual function that has declined due to age.[48]

While there have not been human studies on the subject yet, it can't hurt to add a sprinkle of cinnamon to your meals or drinks as a natural aphrodisiac.

62. EASE ARTHRITIC PAIN

Arthritis is a commonly misunderstood issue—it's often perceived as "a disease for old people," but it's actually a term referring to joint pain or disease. According to the Arthritis Foundation, there are over a hundred types of arthritis and arthritis-related conditions. These can be simplified into four main types of arthritis, all characterized by joint stiffness, swelling, and pain:[49]

1. **Degenerative Arthritis:** This is the most common type of arthritis. It occurs when cartilage wears away and bone begins to rub against bone, causing swelling, pain, and other typical arthritis symptoms.

2. **Inflammatory Arthritis:** This occurs when the immune system mistakes healthy joints for something dangerous and attacks them with inflammation, causing joint pain and erosion.

3. **Infectious Arthritis:** When something outside the body (like a fungus, virus, or bacterium) enters the joint, this can trigger inflammation, resulting in this type of arthritis.

4. **Metabolic Arthritis:** To understand this type of arthritis, we first need to understand what "uric acid" is. Uric acid is a natural waste product that is produced when you digest foods with purines (chemical compounds found in foods like beer, organ meats, and seafood). If your body has a high uric acid level and isn't able to lower it quickly enough, the acid can build up, causing joint pain.

The bottom line—there are different causes of the joint pain that characterize arthritis, but the erosion of cartilage and increased inflammation are common denominators.

That's why cinnamon is helpful for easing pain—researchers have found cinnamon slows down the breakdown of bones.[50] It also has anti-inflammatory properties, which is especially helpful for inflammatory and infectious arthritis.[51] Finally, the spice has antioxidant properties from the cinnamaldehyde and cinnamic acid it contains. This helps fight free radicals that damage cells in your body, lowering inflammation.[52]

63. HELP PREVENT NEURODEGENERATIVE DISEASES

Neurodegenerative diseases, such as Parkinson's and Alzheimer's, affect about 50 million Americans each year.[53] Having a family member or close friend who suffers from a neurodegenerative disease can be devastating—as their nervous system gradually begins to lose more and more cells, their memory, speech, and ability to perform tasks can begin to deteriorate as well.

In many cases, it's hard to pinpoint the exact cause of neurodegenerative diseases. Scientists theorize some diseases can be attributed to environmental factors (such as heavy metals, like copper, selenium, zinc, lead, and mercury), while other diseases, like Alzheimer's, can be predicted by four known risk factors (age, familial history, the presence of Down syndrome, and the apolipoprotein E4 allele).[54]

To understand how cinnamon can help prevent diseases like Parkinson's and Alzheimer's, we have to first understand how the brain changes when these diseases occur.

Let's look first at Alzheimer's disease. In your brain, nerve cells called neurons are supported by microtubules. These are structures that help guide nutrients from the cell body to the axon and dendrites (structures at either end of the cell body). There is also a protein called tau, which binds to and helps stabilize microtubules in healthy neurons.

In brains affected by Alzheimer's, however, the tau detaches from the microtubules and sticks to other tau molecules. This causes a neurofibrillary tangle and blocks the neuron's transport system so it cannot communicate properly.[55]

A recent study found cinnamon inhibits this buildup of tau molecules. It's important to note that cinnamon (used as a water-based extract of Ceylon cinnamon in this particular study) did not affect tau's ability to perform its regular functions; instead, it only prevented tau aggregation.[56]

Parkinson's disease is the second most common neurodegenerative disease in the US (after Alzheimer's). It's characterized by the loss of nerve cells in the substantia nigra, the part of the brain responsible for producing dopamine.

Dopamine is a neurotransmitter that acts as a messenger between the brain and the nervous system—specifically the parts that control body movements.[57] When too many nerve cells in the substantia nigra die (symptoms are typically seen at 80 percent loss), the body's control center starts to malfunction, causing the slow, jerky movements that characterize Parkinson's.

Studies have found ground cinnamon helps halt the progression of Parkinson's because, when ingested orally, it is metabolized into sodium benzoate. This then enters the brain, protecting neurons, normalizing neurotransmitters, and improving motor functions.[58] Although the study showed both Ceylon cinnamon and cassia cinnamon were effective, Ceylon proved to be more effective because of its high coumarin content.

There is currently no cure for neurodegenerative diseases, but the daily use of cinnamon is a hope and can be a preventative measure for those suffering from or for those wishing to avoid these diseases.

NUTRITION

BEAUTY

HEALTH

HOME

64. HELP PREVENT OSTEOPOROSIS

Osteoporosis is a disease that impacts your bones; either your body loses too much bone or makes too little bone. The word itself means "porous bone," which reflects how the bone looks when under a microscope—the naturally occurring holes in osteoporotic bones are much larger than normal. This causes bones to be less dense, more brittle, and weaker than healthy bones.

Osteoporosis impacts about 54 million Americans, especially the elderly. About one in every two women, and up to one in four men, older than fifty are at risk for breaking a bone due to osteoporosis.[59]

Cinnamaldehyde, the aldehyde that gives cinnamon its signature flavor, has been identified to reduce osteoclast-like cell formations.[60] Osteoclasts are bone-reabsorbing cells and are the culprits of many instances of bone loss.[61] Thus, the reduction of osteoclast function and formation means cinnamon can help prevent osteoporosis.

To help build healthy, strong bones, you can eat bone-strengthening foods that are rich in calcium, like milk and nuts, and combine them with cinnamon for an extra bone-boosting meal or snack.

65. EASE NAUSEA

Nausea, or feeling the need to vomit, can be caused by a variety of factors: food poisoning, pregnancy, pain, ulcers, overeating, chemotherapy, medication, toxins, motion sickness, and diseases affecting the brain, throat, stomach, and other organs. It is considered to be a form of biological protection, warning you not to ingest something toxic.[62]

No matter the cause, nausea is deeply uncomfortable and inconvenient. Cinnamon can help ease nausea both from its aroma and by ingestion. The scent of cinnamon helps ease and calm the nerves, which is helpful because nausea is typically accompanied by other types of pain.[63] Because it is also an antibacterial and antifungal agent, it helps kill any toxins in your body that may be caused by bacteria. Cinnamon bark has also been used to treat nausea in chemotherapy patients.[64] For women who suffer from dysmenorrhea, cinnamon has been shown to reduce both the severity of nausea and the frequency of vomiting in association to a severe menstrual cycle.[65]

So the next time you feel nauseous, brew some cinnamon tea and sip on it slowly to help ease symptoms.

66. SOOTHE A STIFF NECK

If you've woken up with neck soreness or a neck so stiff you're unable to move your head, you know how annoying it is—not to mention a little scary. You may go about the rest of your day unable to turn your head too much to either side.

Not to worry. There are a few steps you can take to relieve the stiffness in your neck. It is advised to do them in the morning or when you first experience the pain, so you can address the problem as quickly as possible.

First, apply a warm compress (you can use a towel and warm water—bonus points if you add soothing essential oils!) to the spot. Heat is helpful in relaxing muscles and helps bring blood flow to the area. Second, while you're sitting with the warm compress, sip on an herbal tea made with 1/4 teaspoon ground cinnamon (or one whole cinnamon stick) and 1/4 teaspoon ground turmeric (or one 1-inch piece of fresh turmeric) mixed with 8 ounces of hot water. Both spices have significant anti-inflammatory properties, and turmeric has the added benefit of soothing muscle soreness.[66]

Repeat this process as many times as you need to alleviate the stiffness (or as many times as you have time for). It can also be a good way to wind down at the end of the day, before you go to bed.

67. PREVENT AND TREAT UTIs

More than 7 million people visit hospitals each year for treatment of urinary tract infections (UTIs).[67] These infections are typically caused by the bacterium Uropathogenic Escherichia coli (UPEC), which causes irritation in your bladder and urethra. UTIs usually result in symptoms like burning or even pain when urinating and feeling the strong need to use the bathroom often but only producing a few drops of urine.[68]

Women are more likely to get UTIs than men (about 60 percent of women get one in their lifetime compared to about 12 percent of men) because of their shorter urethra—meaning bacteria have a shorter distance to travel.

The typical treatment for UTIs is a course of antibiotics to kill the problematic bacteria. However, in the case of repeated UTIs, the bacteria may develop a resistance to the antibiotics, presenting the need for an alternative treatment.

Cinnamon can help you avoid and treat UTIs because of its anti-bacterial and antifungal properties—trans-cinnamaldehyde, the active compound in cinnamon, has been seen to decrease UPEC populations in the body.[69]

The best measure is a preventative measure, so we recommend adding cinnamon to your meals. Consuming cranberry juice and adequate amounts of water are also recommended by the Urology Care Foundation as preventative measures.[70]

68. AID IN WEIGHT LOSS

People ate half a grapefruit with cinnamon sprinkled on top as a popular diet breakfast in the 1930s,[71] but it turns out they were actually onto something. A 2006 *J Med Food* study found grapefruit reduced insulin resistance and helped the test group lose weight.[72]

But don't forget the cinnamon! This spice is similarly effective in reducing insulin resistance. The Human Nutrition Center at Tufts University reported cinnamon, even in small daily doses, increases insulin's capacity to metabolize blood sugar. That means it can be used to help reduce hunger, curb sugar cravings, and ease the effects of diabetes—all of which are useful in losing weight.[73]

NUTRITION

BEAUTY

HEALTH

HOME

Why does insulin resistance matter? you might be asking yourself. Well, if you've ever tried to lose weight by sticking to the perfect diet and exercise plan but found that the pounds just weren't coming off, insulin resistance might be the culprit.

When your body is insulin resistant, it means the food you eat isn't being properly converted into the energy you need to fuel your body. That's because insulin is the hormone your body uses to convert food (like carbs) into glucose (sugar your cells can use) and move glucose from your blood into your cells. In cases of insulin resistance, your body is no longer sensitive to insulin, meaning it takes more and more insulin to move glucose into your cells. When your body can no longer produce enough insulin and too much glucose is left in your blood, you become diabetic. Because there is nowhere else for the glucose to go, your body turns it into fat as a way to store it for later.[74]

Cinnamon has a two-pronged benefit here: It helps reduce insulin resistance, as we mentioned earlier, *and* it can potentially help your fat cells burn energy.[75] That means glucose is less likely to be stored as fat in your body and existing fat cells may enter fat-burning mode with the consumption of cinnamon.

So here's to a breakfast topped with cinnamon, whether that's cinnamon oatmeal or your typical cinnamon-dusted grapefruit!

69. CURB CRAVINGS

Sugar cravings are real—studies have shown that sugar can be addicting and can even act as a gateway to alcohol use.[76] These days, though, sugar seems to be in *everything*, even foods you think are savory.

The easiest way to lower your sugar intake is to focus on cooking your own food, because many processed foods have added sugar or sugar substitutes in them. To make the transition a little easier, you can use cinnamon as a sugar substitute. Because cinnamon naturally tastes sweet, you can use it to replace some of the sugar you would normally add to a drink or a food (for example, if you typically use one spoonful of sugar in your coffee, you can add a pinch of cinnamon and a half spoonful of sugar). Cinnamon makes a great addition to such items as coffee, oatmeal, yogurt, and even baked goods.

There is also science behind why cinnamon can help curb cravings—naturally occurring compounds in cinnamon help improve insulin sensitivity.[77] This is important because if you have insulin resistance, glucose can't properly enter your cells. Your body then starts to crave sugar and carbs as a response.[78]

70. REDUCE CHOLESTEROL

According to the Center of Disease Control (CDC), about one in three adults in America has high cholesterol.[79] But what does high cholesterol mean and why is it bad?

Like we covered in the "Boost Heart Health" section, there are two types of cholesterol:

1. **"Bad" cholesterol:** LDL cholesterol, which contributes to fat buildup in your arteries.
2. **"Good" cholesterol:** HDL cholesterol, which carries LDL cholesterol away from your arteries and back into your liver, thus preventing too much fatty buildup.

Unlike other "diseases," you won't feel any particular symptoms if you have high LDL cholesterol, which is why doctors typically check your lipid levels during physical exams. Lipids are fat-like molecules found in your bloodstream. Cholesterol and triglycerides are both examples of a lipid.[80]

It's important to maintain low LDL cholesterol levels to avoid heart disease and stroke. This can be managed by living a healthy, active lifestyle: make smart eating choices, exercise regularly, limit alcohol consumption, cut out smoking, and maintain a healthy weight.

If you already have high cholesterol levels, you can bring those levels down by doing the things listed above . . . and getting a little help from cinnamon. Cinnamon has been shown to reduce LDL cholesterol levels in people with type II diabetes by up to 27 percent over the course of a forty-day trial.[81] In addition, a 2017 review compiled thirteen studies on cinnamon's effect on lipid levels. Researchers concluded cinnamon "significantly lowered total cholesterol, LDL cholesterol, and triglyceride levels."[82]

For those struggling with high cholesterol levels, adding cinnamon to your daily diet can be a tool to help you bring your cholesterol levels down.

71. PAIN RELIEVER

Before the invention of modern painkillers, people used natural remedies created from herbs. For centuries, herbs like St. John's wort, ginseng, and cinnamon have been used topically and orally to help relieve pain.

While nonsteroidal anti-inflammatory drugs (NSAID) have become the go-to medicine for pain relief, there may be cases when it is unwise to use over-the-counter drugs (such as ibuprofen or Advil). For example, in instances of the coronavirus (COVID-19), using NSAIDs may actually worsen the disease and the Food and Drug Administration (FDA) has recommended against the use of these drugs.[83] In such cases, or for those who prefer a natural remedy, cinnamon may act as a safer substitute that will still help relieve pain.

Cinnamon is an effective pain reliever because it reacts with prostaglandin, which is a group of lipids that are created in parts of your body where tissue is damaged or infected—meaning they deal with illness and injury. Recent studies have found cinnamon to be nearly as effective as NSAID ibuprofen in cases of dysmenorrhea (menstrual cramps).[84] Cinnamon also creates a muscle-relaxing effect.

72. EASE PMS SYMPTOMS, ESPECIALLY DYSMENORRHEA

Dysmenorrhea, or menstrual cramps, is a common PMS (premenstrual syndrome) symptom for many women who have regular menstrual cycles. In fact, it's estimated that 20 percent of women will have dysmenorrhea so severe at some point in their life that it will impact their daily activities.[85] These cramps come from your uterus and can be categorized into two types:

NUTRITION

BEAUTY

HEALTH

HOME

1. **Primary dysmenorrhea:** Pain that does not have an organic cause. This is the type most women have.
2. **Secondary dysmenorrhea:** Pain that is associated with a pathological condition, like endometriosis or ovarian cysts.

If you smoke, have long periods, or start your period at an early age, you may have an increased chance of getting primary dysmenorrhea. Many women learn to accept these as a given side effect of having a period and treat them with over-the-counter medications like ibuprofen.

Cinnamon has been shown in multiple studies to help relieve menstrual symptoms. Not only does it reduce the amount of menstrual blood and the frequency and severity of nausea and vomiting, but it also reduces overall pain.[86] In addition, cinnamon was shown to significantly reduce both the severity *and* duration of pain during the menstrual cycle, with results almost as effective as ibuprofen.[87]

The next time you feel PMS symptoms—especially cramps—coming on, get yourself a warm compress, sip some cinnamon tea, and sprinkle cinnamon generously on your food to help reduce the pain so you can live your life unbothered by the pesky effects of PMS.

73. HELP TREAT POLYCYSTIC OVARIAN SYNDROME

PCOS, or polycystic ovarian syndrome, is a hormonal disorder that affects 6–12 percent of women of reproductive age in the

United States, making it one of the most common causes of female infertility in the US.[88]

The causes for PCOS are not certain, but elevated androgen levels, excess weight, and a family history of PCOS or type II diabetes are thought to be contributing factors. Insulin resistance can both be a contributing factor and a symptom; in both cases, it is beneficial to lower insulin resistance.

This is where cinnamon comes in. Cinnamon can help lower insulin resistance; it's been shown to help in studies with type II diabetes patients and on a trial study of women with PCOS. The latter study found cinnamon helped treat PCOS by reducing the level of insulin-like growth factor-I (IGF-I) and increase the level of insulin-like growth factor-binding protein 1 (IGFBP 1).[89]

Cinnamon has thus been demonstrated to serve as a potential therapeutic agent for treating PCOS because it downregulates testosterone and insulin.

74. BOOST YOUR IMMUNE SYSTEM

Your immune system is your body's first line of defense against invaders—germs, viruses, infections, bacteria, disease, etc. A healthy immune system is not only able to identify your body's normal cells, but it's also able to identify unhealthy or dangerous cells using natural danger cues.[90]

Your immune system cells all develop from your bone marrow, but they mature via different parts in your body, including your skin, bloodstream, thymus, lymphatic system, and spleen. As you age, your immune system starts to decline, which is why elderly people are more at risk for disease and why they may have a harder time fighting these diseases off.

That's why having a strong immune system is so important: It helps protect you from sickness and makes you less susceptible to severe symptoms even if you do fall sick.

There are various ways to strengthen your immune system. First, maintain a healthy lifestyle. This means no smoking and eating a diet rich in a variety of fruits and vegetables. Like the healthy lifestyle tenets for avoiding high cholesterol, the other pillars of maintaining a strong immune system are exercising regularly, getting adequate sleep, drinking alcohol in moderation, and maintaining a healthy weight.

Second, keep your stress levels low. Scientists hypothesize high levels of stress can take a huge toll on your immune system; we know high stress levels can impact everything from your weight, to your quality of sleep, to your mood. While it is hard to pin down stress in a laboratory setting, it is generally recommended that you reduce your stress levels.

In times of high immune stress, like cold and flu season or a global pandemic, it can be helpful to bolster your immune system with herbs and spices. Cinnamon is a particularly useful one to use—not only is cinnamon full of antioxidants, but it has also been shown to activate the immune system.[91] There's a reason why cinnamon is so enticing in the winter—that's when cold and flu season is generally at its peak and when your body needs the extra immunity boost. Try this homemade syrup to help keep your immune system strong.

GINGER ELDERBERRY IMMUNITY-BOOSTING CINNAMON SYRUP

1 bottle elderberry syrup (or 1 cup dried/fresh elderberries; however, if you use fresh, triple the water and honey)

1 cup water

2 cinnamon sticks

1/2 knob of ginger

1/4 cup honey

1. In a small pot, combine all ingredients except the honey.
2. Cover and simmer for 30 minutes to an hour.
3. Remove from the heat and strain through a cheesecloth to get the syrup.
4. Add honey and mix well.
5. Pour into a glass bottle and use a spoonful or two each day, or as needed.

75. HELP PREVENT PARASITES

The word *parasite* can seem scary—the idea of another living organism feeding on you, your family, or your pets can be a lot to handle. It's a problem that has endured through time. The first written record of parasites in humans was in Egypt between 3000 and 400 BCE. Since then, ancient Chinese, Arab, Greek, and Indian physicians have all written about diseases and symptoms that were likely caused by parasites. Throughout Earth's history, over 370 species of parasites have been discovered; however, most of these are rare. Today, only about ninety common species of parasites remain, most of which are located in the tropics.[92]

As modern medicine develops, parasites are becoming more drug resistant as their self-defense mechanisms kick into gear. To make matters worse, it is difficult to figure out whether you have a parasite without doctor-performed tests. If you suspect you or someone you know may have a parasite, it's best to visit a doctor, but here is one remedy you can take in the meantime. It also helps serve as a preventative measure.

Essential oils can be immensely helpful due to their natural healing properties. Cinnamon oil especially can help prevent larvae from moving to different parts of the body—it ranked the most effective out of all the botanicals it was tested against. It can also even help kill the larvae.[93] Clove essential oil contains a powerful compound called eugenol, which can help eradicate pathogens in the gut.[94] If you think you have parasites, mix 1 drop of cinnamon essential oil, 1 drop of clove essential oil, 1 tablespoon of honey (or to taste), and 8 ounces of water or ginger tea. Drink up to two times a day until you visit your doctor for a blood test and to see if further treatment is necessary.

CHAPTER 4

FOR THE HOME-IMPROVEMENT MASTER IN YOU

NUTRITION

BEAUTY

HEALTH

HOME

76. DOG FOOD

While your dog may not be able to eat some human spices—like cayenne, black pepper, or even too much salt—Ceylon cinnamon is safe for dogs in small amounts because it has lower coumarin levels.

The human benefits of cinnamon also benefit dogs: it makes their food taste better, warms them from the inside out, helps their digestion, helps disinfect their food to reduce the risk of bacterial infections, promotes bone and cartilage development, helps with arthritis relief, and helps maintain a healthy weight by stabilizing blood sugar levels.[1] Use the chart below to help determine how much cinnamon per serving is safe for your pet.

Pet's Weight	Amount of Cinnamon Powder per Meal
<10 pounds	1/16 teaspoon
10–20 pounds	1/16–1/8 teaspoon
21–50 pounds	1/8–1/2 teaspoon
51–100 pounds	1/4–3/4 teaspoon
>100 pounds	3/4–1 teaspoon

You can start by adding the appropriate amount of cinnamon to your dog's dry or wet food with some warm water, or you can try this cinnamon dog food recipe:

PEANUT BUTTER PUMPKIN SPICE TREATS

3/4 cup coconut flour

1/2 cup organic canned pumpkin

1/4 cup sugar-, salt-, and oil-free natural peanut butter

1/4 cup honey

1/2 very-ripe banana

3 tablespoons plain Greek yogurt

2 teaspoons cinnamon

1. Combine all ingredients together and roll into bite-size balls.
2. Store in the fridge and give to your pet as desired once per day.

77. FUNGICIDE PLANT SPRAY

Cinnamon isn't just an antifungal for humans—it's an antifungal for plants as well; cinnamon essential oil has been shown to be effective against a multitude of plant diseases caused by fungi, such as dry bubble, dollar spot, and pitch canker disease.[2]

Unlike regular fungicides, using organic cinnamon to kill fungus is 100 percent organic and chemical-free. You don't have to worry about ingesting any toxins if you choose to harvest and eat these plants from your garden. It's easy to make a cinnamon fungicide spray—all you need is cinnamon essential oil and water!

CINNAMON FUNGICIDE PLANT SPRAY

24 ounces water

4 drops cinnamon essential oil

1. Combine ingredients in a spray bottle and shake vigorously.

NUTRITION

BEAUTY

HEALTH

HOME

2. Spray directly on affected plants and soil once per day until the affected area gets better.

Note: This can be used as a preventative measure as well—spray on the soil to prevent fungus from growing. Alternatively, you can sprinkle cinnamon powder directly on the soil.

....

78. PLANT HEALER

You know humans can have open wounds and need time to heal, but did you know your plants can too? And just like human wounds can get infected, so can plant wounds. Help heal plant wounds quickly and prevent fungus from growing by sprinkling cinnamon powder on the wound.[3]

....

79. SEEDLING PROTECTANT

When cultivating plants, there are two options:

1. **Direct seeding:** Growing a plant straight from the seeds.
2. **Transplanting seedlings:** Taking cuttings from an existing plant and transplanting them in new soil.

Some plants are easier to grow as direct seeds. These include beans, squashes, pumpkins, watermelons, plants with long taproots (including carrots and beets), and root vegetables (including parsnips and turnips). This is because these plants typically grow quickly and do not do well with transplanting. Other vegetables— such as cruciferous vegetables (broccoli, Brussels sprouts, and

NUTRITION

cauliflower), collard greens, eggplants, and peppers—are better transplanted as seedlings.

Whether you're growing your plants from seeds or transplanting them, you'll want to protect the plants from damping off. "Damping off" is the term used for a new seedling's sudden death. Contrary to popular belief, damping off is not a single disease, but rather a result of a group of diseases, including fungal diseases and mold.[4]

Once one plant has signs of damping off, the symptoms can spread quickly. Remove the infected seedling immediately and take preventative measures on the rest of the plants. There is no cure for damping off, which means the best method is prevention. Cinnamon can be used in two ways to help prevent damping off:

1. **Mist your seedlings with a cinnamon brew.** Brew cinnamon tea (1 bag 100% cinnamon tea (or 1 cinnamon stick) to 8 ounces of water). Once cooled, put it in a spray bottle and use spray onto your seedlings.

2. **Sprinkle ground cinnamon on your plants.** You can sprinkle the surface of the soil with ground cinnamon.

Cinnamon is effective because of its antifungal properties, meaning it inhibits the growth of mold and fungus. In addition, cinnamon water has a stimulating effect on tomato plant growth.[5]

BEAUTY

80. PLANT ROOTING AGENT

If you've ever wanted a new plant but didn't want to grow it from a seed every time, using existing plant cuttings is a great option.

HEALTH

HOME

It cuts down on the growth time—plus you get the added benefit of certainty. You don't have to wonder if your seed is ever going to sprout; the plant is already above the ground when you transplant it. You are essentially cloning your old plant and creating a new one.

Rooting hormones are typically used in transplanting. They help stimulate the growth of a plant cutting and increase the chances of your plant surviving. Most commonly, rooting hormones are used for ornamental plants and succulents.[6]

If you don't have time to run to the home improvement store for a rooting hormone, or simply want to save some money, you can use cinnamon in place of a store-bought rooting hormone. Cinnamon will help prevent disease and infection from reaching your plant, helping it grow strong and healthy. Simply wet your cutting in water and roll it in ground cinnamon before planting it.

81. ANT REPELLANT

Have an ant problem? Although these insects may not be dangerous, they *are* quite annoying. Good news: This common household problem can be easily solved with the cinnamon powder sitting in your pantry.

The compounds in cinnamon activate an ion channel in the ants' antennae and send a signal that there are harmful conditions nearby.[7] This causes the ants to stay away from the substance.

Sprinkle cinnamon directly on ant tracks and nests and you'll see them start to stay away from those places. You can use it in the garden or in your home to help ward off these pests.

82. MOSQUITO LARVAE EXTERMINATOR

Mosquitos are pesky insects that can carry a number of diseases, including the dangerous West Nile and Zika viruses, as well as malaria.[8] That means the bites aren't just annoying; they can potentially be harmful as well.

One good way to avoid mosquitos is to make sure there are no larvae hiding in or near your home. Mosquitoes typically like laying eggs in or near standing (still) water. If you have a pond or frequent puddles in your yard, it's more likely that you'll have a mosquito larvae problem.

To nip this problem in the bud, you can use cinnamon essential oil to get rid of the mosquito larvae. Cinnamon was found to be effective in killing both wild and lab-bred mosquito larvae.[9] The higher the dosage, the more larvae were exterminated.

To create your own mosquito larvae repellent, use 4 drops of cinnamon essential oil per 8 ounces of water for maximum efficiency.

83. AUTUMN-SCENTED ROOM SPRAY

Each season seems to have its own specific aroma, and nothing says fall like a cozy cinnamon scent. This combination of essential oils evokes a warm yet forest-y feel. With its all-natural ingredients,

NUTRITION

BEAUTY

HEALTH

HOME

it's a spray you'll want to use over and over again in the autumn months.

The main component is cinnamon essential oil, but you can omit some of the essential oils if you don't have them. The witch hazel in the recipe helps the water and essential oils stay mixed together.[10]

AUTUMN-SCENTED ROOM SPRAY

8 ounces water

8 ounces witch hazel (unscented)

20 drops cinnamon essential oil

10 drops clove essential oil

5 drops vanilla essential oil

5 drops cardamom essential oil

5 drops ginger essential oil

5 drops frankincense essential oil

5 drops pine or spruce essential oil

1. Combine in a spray bottle and shake vigorously to mix.
2. Spritz around your home as desired to evoke a relaxing autumn evening.

84. CINNAMON STICK PLACE CARDS

A way to instantly make any dinner party feel more fancy is to create place cards for your guests. It's also great if you want to control who is sitting where—this can help avoid arguments, spark interesting conversations, inspire new connections, and more. Even if it's just for an extended family holiday dinner, creating place settings can level up the occasion from "a big meal" to "a family feast."

Buying place settings can be expensive, especially if you have a lot of place settings to get. This is where cinnamon comes in! You can use cinnamon sticks to make festive, budget friendly, and great-smelling place settings. This works especially well for fall and winter weddings, as well as Thanksgiving, Christmas Eve, and Christmas dinners.

CINNAMON STICK PLACE CARDS

Cinnamon sticks of similar lengths (one for every person who needs a place card)

Thick, high-quality paper (white is recommended)

Permanent marker, calligraphy pen, or any other thick marker

1. Lay a cinnamon stick along the edge of the paper. Use a ruler to mark the paper one inch shorter than the cinnamon stick.
2. Turn the ruler vertical and make a mark 2.5 to 3 inches down.
3. Cut the paper to the dimensions you marked on the paper. Use this as a template for the other cards. You can also use a paper cutter, for a more precise and faster cut, or purchase precut cards.
4. Once the cards are cut out, write in the names.
5. Slide the bottom of the card into the crack in the cinnamon stick.

85. CINNAMON CANDLES

Before electricity was invented, candles were the primary way people got light. For five thousand years, candles have been made in a variety of ways; Romans used rolled papyrus, the Chinese used rolled paper tubes with rice paper wicks, and Indians used the fruit of the cinnamon tree, which they boiled.[11]

These days, we can get light at the flick of a switch, but candles remain a way for us to instill a sense of coziness in our homes or a sense of romance at the dinner table. Some people even use candles after sundown as a way to avoid artificial lights, which have been shown to affect circadian rhythm and sleep cycles.[12]

Candles are actually easy to make yourself if you have the time and the ingredients. With this natural DIY method, you get a clean-burning smell that won't give you an artificial scent–induced headache.

CINNAMON VANILLA COCONUT OIL CANDLE

8 ounces beeswax
1/2 cup coconut oil
25 drops cinnamon essential oil
20 drops clove essential oil
10 drops vanilla essential oil
5 drops cedar or sandalwood essential oil
Candle wick (thick twine or string)
Crushed cinnamon sticks (optional)

1. Use a double boiler to melt the wax. Remove from the heat once the wax is completely melted. (You can also use a candy thermometer to monitor the heat—once it reaches 150°F, remove from the heat. The temperature may continue to rise—that's normal.)

2. Pour in the coconut oil and combine thoroughly.

3. Add the essential oils. You can add more—if you prefer a stronger scent—or less—if you want a milder scent.

4. Let the wax cool for 3 to 5 minutes, or until it reaches about 160°F.

5. While the wax is cooling, measure your wick. Cut the string until it's slightly longer than the length of a heat-resistant glass jar.

6. Tie one end of the wick around a long object (I recommend a pencil or chopstick).

7. Place the long object lengthwise on the top of the jar so the wick hangs down into the jar. If the wick touches the bottom, trim it until it hangs about a quarter of an inch above the bottom.

8. Pour the cooled wax into the jar slowly. Make sure the wick is centered as you pour—you may need to adjust it from time to time. Stop pouring when the wax is about one inch below the opening of your jar.

9. If you want to decorate the top of your candle with the crushed cinnamon sticks, wait for 10–15 minutes so the top layer of the candle can harden. Then, press the chopped cinnamon sticks gently into the wax.

10. Allow the candle to dry for a day or two, then cut the wick down and burn as desired.

86. CINNAMON-SCENTED PINECONES

Pinecones have become a symbol of the holidays and represent the changing seasons. You can see them on the ground by pine trees, in holiday wreaths, scented and sold in bags in stores, and much more.

As the weather starts to get colder and holiday decorations start to come up, creating your own scented pinecones is an easy and fun way to create a cozy atmosphere in your house. It's an activity you can involve the whole family in—from gathering the pinecones on a walk outside to shaking the bag to imbue the pinecones with scent.

Cinnamon essential oil is the key scent in these DIY scented pinecones. It not only creates the sweet-smelling aroma that screams "warm and cozy," but it can also help improve your memory—an extra bonus.[13]

CINNAMON-SCENTED PINECONES

20-30 pinecones, depending on size (if you buy them instead of gathering them, you can skip directly to step 4)

20 drops cinnamon essential oil

10 drops clove essential oil

5 drops vanilla essential oil

5 drops cedar essential oil

1. If you collected pinecones from outside, soak them in a large bowl full of water for an hour. Place a plate or another object on top of the pinecones to keep them from floating to the top.

2. Line a baking sheet with foil or parchment paper. Spread the pinecones on the sheet and bake at 200°F for about 30 minutes.

3. Let the pinecones cool until they're at room temperature.

4. Transfer the pinecones to a gallon-size Ziploc bag. Depending on how many pinecones you have and how big they are, you may have to use more than one bag.

5. Sprinkle the essential oils into the bag (the amounts above are for one bag of pinecones). Feel free to swap out any essential oils you don't have for ones that you do.

6. Seal the bag and shake to distribute the essential oils evenly.

7. Let the pinecones sit for one to two weeks so the smell layers in completely.

8. Remove the pinecones from the bag and place them in a bowl for a woodsy, holiday-inspired scent.

87. HOMEMADE CLEANING SPRAY

Some of my earliest memories of my mother cleaning in the kitchen involved a giant bottle of white vinegar. I'd wrinkle my nose and run away (literally) because of the smell, but as I grew older and had a place of my own, I began to appreciate how effective white vinegar can be at cleaning household messes. It's a natural alternative to store-bought, chemical-laden cleaners and can effectively strip surfaces of dirt, mildew, and bacteria.[14]

Fortunately, this homemade cleaning spray uses cinnamon to help mask the strong scent of white vinegar. It also acts as an antibacterial agent; cinnamon essential oil has been shown to fight bacteria, especially foodborne pathogens like *E. coli*.[15]

This spray is best used in the kitchen—it can be used on cutting boards, countertops, the kitchen table, and even the floor.

HOMEMADE CINNAMON CLEANING SPRAY

20 drops cinnamon essential oil

8 ounces distilled water

8 ounces white vinegar

1. Combine all ingredients in a spray bottle and shake to combine.
2. Use on surfaces as needed. It's recommended to let the spray sit for about 5 minutes before wiping off.

88. CAR FRESHENER

Getting into your car should be a peaceful experience, not a nauseating one. Unfortunately, because your car is likely sealed up most of the time when it's parked in the sun or garage, odors can quickly develop and linger.

These odors can come from mildew, mold, smoke, sweat, food, dirty clothes, pets, or a musty air filter.[16] It can make your drive uncomfortable—for you and any passengers you might have.

Typical car air fresheners try to mask the scent, but oftentimes they result in an overpowering, headache-inducing artificial smell. Use cinnamon to help freshen the scent of—and even help clean—your car. There are a few ways you can use cinnamon to help freshen up your car:

1. Glue cotton balls or pom-poms to a clothespin. Add one drop of cinnamon essential oil to each cotton ball/pom-pom. Clip to your car's air vents.

2. Mix 1/2 a cup of baking soda and 20 drops of cinnamon essential oil in a Mason jar. Poke holes in the lid—so the scent can diffuse out—and place in your cup holder.

3. Fill a cheesecloth or sachet with cinnamon sticks and tie to your rearview mirror.

4. Buy a car essential oil diffuser; add enough water to fill the diffuser and 1 drop of cinnamon essential oil per ounce of water. If you prefer a stronger scent, feel free to add more essential oil.

5. Combine 4 tablespoons of baking soda and 4 drops of cinnamon essential oil in a small dish. Sprinkle the mixture on your

car floor and seats (if fabric); leave on for 15 minutes and then
vacuum up.

6. Add a few drops of cinnamon essential oil on top of the car
filter for fresh-smelling air when you turn on the AC or heat.

89. CARPET DEODORIZER

Whether you have a pet or some musty-smelling carpets (life happens), there is an easy solution to get fresher smelling carpets—one
that has been used by homeowners for years.

Baking soda is a proven odor absorber—it goes down past the
surface layer of the carpet to truly absorb and neutralize odors.[17]
Once it's had time to soak up the smells, you can vacuum it all up,
leaving you with fresh-smelling carpets!

This homemade deodorizer combines the odor-absorbing
properties of baking soda with the antibacterial properties of cinnamon to create a product that will not only make your rugs and
carpets smell better, but also help prevent bacterial growth in the
future.

CITRUS CINNAMON CARPET DEODORIZER

1 cup baking soda
20 drops grapefruit essential oil
1 teaspoon ground cinnamon

1. Combine all ingredients in a Mason jar.
2. Close the lid and shake vigorously to combine.
3. Sprinkle liberally on carpets as needed. Allow to sit for 20
minutes.
4. Vacuum up and enjoy the fresh scent of your carpets!

90. CINNAMON DIFFuSER

The scent of cinnamon can help boost your mood and help you concentrate better, making it the perfect scent to diffuse in your home.[18]

Diffusers help disperse the scent of essential oils into the air, filling it with the benefits and scent of the essential oils. There are a few ways you can diffuse scent throughout your space. The easiest is to use the lights you have in your home and some cinnamon essential oil. All you have to do is add a drop of cinnamon essential oil to the surface of your light bulb. Once you turn the lights on, you'll smell cinnamon!

If you have an essential oil diffuser already, simply add 3 drops of cinnamon essential oil per 4 ounces of water. If you want to combine scents, you can use clove, cedar, or vanilla essential oils as well.

Finally, you can make a classic cinnamon reed diffuser (directions below). It's a great way to recycle any old jars and use up cinnamon sticks and orange peels.

HOMEMADE CINNAMON REED DiFFUSER

Peels from 1 orange, thinly sliced
2 whole cinnamon sticks
2 sprigs fresh rosemary
3/4 cup water
1/4 cup rubbing alcohol
10 drops cinnamon essential oil
5 drops rosemary essential oil
5 drops orange essential oil
10-12 bamboo skewers

NUTRITION

BEAUTY

HEALTH

HOME

1. Add orange peels, cinnamon sticks, and rosemary to a small glass jar or bottle (the smaller the opening, the better; reusing old oil bottles are great because they have a pour spout).
2. Add water and rubbing alcohol to the jar. If the jar is too small, simply use less liquid, but keep the same proportions.
3. Add essential oils to the jar and gently stir to incorporate the liquids.
4. Stick the bamboo skewers into the jar. If your jar has a spout, put it in before adding the bamboo skewers.
5. That's it! Change the liquid every two to three weeks to prevent mold from building up from the herbs, spices, and orange peels in the liquid.

91. MoSQuiTo REPELLANT

Mosquito bites can be unbearably itchy and unbelievably annoying. Female mosquitoes bite because they need the blood to develop fertile eggs. They can sense where we are through proteins in their antennae, which latch onto human chemical markers.[19]

Some people get bitten more often than others. While scientists don't know exactly why this happens, a couple of factors seem to be at play. These factors include blood type (type O people, you get bitten more often!), carbon dioxide emissions (via breath), heat emitted, sweat, pregnancy, and genetics.

DEET (N,N-diethyl-meta-toluamide) is a chemical that many insect repellants use to deter mosquitoes.[20] However, there has been speculation about whether this chemical is safe. Whether you're avoiding DEET or prefer to save money by making your own mosquito repellant, you can use the recipe below to stay relatively bite- and itch-free throughout the summer.

This mosquito repellant contains lemon eucalyptus oil, which has been proven to be just as effective and long-lasting as products containing DEET. The addition of cinnamon oil, which has been known to kill mosquitoes, creates a great-smelling, effective repellent.[21]

CINNAMON LEMON EUCALYPTUS MOSQUITO REPELLENT

10 drops cinnamon essential oil
9 milliliters lemon eucalyptus oil (not the essential oil)
3 ounces liquid coconut oil

1.   Combine all ingredients in a bottle. Shake well.
2.   Apply on your body before going outside.

92. PREVENT MOTHS

If you have fur, silk, leather, or wool clothing you don't wear for most of the year, they can be prone to clothes moths. These pests feed on animal fibers, which contain keratin.[22] They're hard to detect because they avoid light and are quite small, but their effects are quite annoying and can wreak havoc on your precious clothes.

While mothballs are a standard way to protect your clothing, they are still an insecticide. The active ingredient in most store-bought mothballs is either naphthalene or paradichlorobenzene, which can turn from solids into toxic vapor.[23]

Cinnamon can be a natural anti-moth solution. Moths dislike the smell of cinnamon, so by placing a few cinnamon sticks in your closet or clothing drawers, you can prevent moths from eating through your sweaters.[24] Vacuum-sealing frequently un-worn clothes is another layer of protection; you can simply place a few cinnamon sticks in your vacuum-sealed bags and your clothes will smell nicely of cinnamon!

93. HOME HUMIDIFIER

Winter months signal the coming of dry skin and chapped lips due to the drier air. This also makes people more susceptible to catching a cold or the flu, because the dry air can weaken your body's defenses.[25]

Humidifiers can help combat this—they add moisture back into the air. However, there are some downsides to electrical humidifiers. The moistness of the humidifier creates a popular breeding ground for bacteria. Because humidifiers impact the air in your house, breathing in the bacteria can cause a whole new host of health problems.

There are a few easy ways to add more humidity to your home. You can use showers to your advantage—they automatically create a lot of humidity! Simply add a few drops of cinnamon essential oil to the shower before you step in and you'll get cinnamon-scented moist air right in your bathroom.

You can also use houseplants—they increase the amount of humidity in your home. Bowls of water also work, although to a lesser effect.

Finally, you can boil water to create homemade air freshener (instructions in the next use) and put a fan by the pot to help circulate the air throughout your home.

94. CINNAMON AIR FRESHENER

When I was growing up, my family never used store-bought air fresheners (my mom claimed they gave her a headache), and now, after too many incidents at friends' houses or stores where the air was heavy with artificial fragrance, neither do I.

Even though air fresheners are prevalent, the magazine *Science Direct* discloses that air fresheners—even ones labeled as "green" and "organic"—can emit potentially hazardous chemicals and can result in migraine headaches. Typically, less than 10 percent of air freshener ingredients are shared with the public, meaning we don't really know what store-bought air fresheners contain.[26]

That's why this stovetop method my mother used to make our house smell cozy is so effective—it's simply made from heating spices and orange peel in boiling water to emit a warm, inviting scent. You can also use this method with a variety of herbs for different scents, like rosemary or lavender, but this cinnamon combination is especially great for fall.

HOMEMADE CINNAMON AIR FRESHENER

4 organic oranges, peeled
6 whole cinnamon sticks
1/8 cup whole cloves
2 tablespoons ground nutmeg
1 tablespoon ground allspice
3 cups water

1. Dehydrate the orange peels using a food dehydrator or oven (if using an oven, bake at 225°F for 30 minutes).

2. Mix the dehydrated peels with the spices.

3. Heat the water in a saucepan or pot until boiling. Bring the heat to a simmer.

4. Add the spices and orange peel mixture.

5. Keep the pan at a simmer for as long as you want to make the air smell fragrant. If you want to reuse, simply add more water.

95. POTPOURRI

Potpourri, which is essentially dried flowers and spices placed in a pot, has been used to freshen rooms since the twelfth century.[27] Nowadays, it's an easy way to decorate your home for fall. It also makes great homemade gifts!

HOMEMADE POTPOURRI

1 orange (I recommend navel or Cara Cara)
12 whole cinnamon sticks
10 whole star anise
10 whole cloves

1. Cut the orange into thin slices (I recommend using a mandolin) and dehydrate using a food dehydrator or oven (if using an oven, bake at 250°F for 2 hours).

2. Combine with the spices.

3. Store in a sealed jar for at least a day to allow the scents to combine.

4. Place in a decorative bowl or jar to give rooms a lovely aroma. They also make great gifts!

5. When the scent begins to fade, place in boiling water and lower to a simmer to wholly use up the product one last time.

NUTRITION

BEAUTY

HEALTH

HOME

96. NATURAL YOGA MAT SPRAY

It's important to keep your yoga mat clean—it can hold sweat and dirt and be a breeding ground for bacteria, especially if you keep it rolled up and in a dark place. Fortunately, it's easy to create a yoga mat spray at home that will help you keep your mat clean without destroying it (mats can be expensive!).

Essential oils mixed with water and witch hazel are all you need. Witch hazel serves as a cleaning agent (you can also use white vinegar in a pinch!). Water will help distill the cleaning agent. The essential oils not only act as scents, but also as antibacterial agents.

Cinnamon and tea tree oil are two of these incredibly potent, bacteria-fighting essential oils.[28] The DIY mat cleaner below not only smells wonderful, but also effectively cleans your mat. And it's gentle enough to use after every practice!

CINNAMON YOGA MAT SPRAY

1/4 cup witch hazel
10 drops cinnamon essential oil
10 drops clove essential oil
10 drops orange essential oil
5 drops eucalyptus essential oil
3 drops tea tree essential oil
6-8 ounces distilled water

1. Combine all ingredients in a spray bottle.
2. Shake well to mix.
3. Spray on your mat as needed. Wipe clean and allow to hang or lay flat to dry.

NUTRITION

BEAUTY

HEALTH

HOME

97. CINNAMON BROOM

Brooms have been used throughout history to sweep and clean houses, but they also served as symbolic representations to ward off evil spirits. Such brooms were called besom brooms and were made of twigs tied to a handle. If you put such a broom in your house with the twigs up, it was thought to protect your home and dispel negative energy.[29]

Today, such brooms are no longer used as a method of cleaning. Rather, they're used for decoration during the fall months. Cinnamon brooms are sold at grocery stores throughout the United States as sweet-scented home decor.

However, grocery store brooms may quickly lose their scent. Instead of replacing it every time the aroma fades, you can revive the broom's cinnamon scent with the following method:

Mix 20 drops of cinnamon essential oil with 2 ounces of olive, avocado, or coconut oil and rub over the broom's bristles. Make sure you're wearing gloves to protect your hands because the essential oil may burn.

This will help refreshen the broom's scent so you can enjoy the cozy cinnamon fragrance all autumn long!

98. DE-STINK STINKY SHOES

Shoes, especially athletic shoes, are great at harboring bacteria. Your feet sweat in them (there are two hundred and fifty thousand sweat glands in your feet!) and your shoes are left to contain all this moisture—up to half a pint each day.[30] Bacteria can then grow on your feet, transferring to your socks and shoes.

And then these shoes are often left in dark lockers or closets— the perfect breeding ground. The first step to eliminating these bacteria is to pull them out into broad sunlight. While the shoes are in the UV rays, make the bacteria-blasting spray below and spray liberally on the shoes to kill the bacteria. The mix of rubbing alcohol, witch hazel, and essential oils helps kill the bacteria in the shoes.

After allowing the shoes to dry for at least two hours in the sun, sprinkle on the odor-eliminating powder below. The baking soda helps neutralize the smell, and the arrowroot powder helps dry up the shoes. Cinnamon essential oil not only helps the shoes smell better, but also provides extra antibacterial protection, meaning the bacteria are less likely to return.[31] You can also use this powder in between wears.

BACTERIA-BLASTING SPRAY

1 ounce witch hazel
1 ounce rubbing alcohol
2 ounces distilled water
6 drops peppermint essential oil
4 drops tea tree essential oil
2 drops eucalyptus essential oil
1 drop rosemary essential oil

1. Fill a spray bottle a quarter of the way with witch hazel.
2. Fill the bottle up to halfway with rubbing alcohol.
3. Fill the remaining half with distilled water.
4. Add the essential oils and mix well.
5. Spray the mixture on your shoes as needed.

ODOR-ELIMINATING SHOE POWDER

1/4 cup baking soda
1/4 cup arrowroot powder
8 drops cinnamon essential oil
5 drops rosemary essential oil
3 drops tea tree essential oil

1. Combine all ingredients in a glass jar and shake to mix.
2. Use on your shoes as needed.

99. HOLIDAY ORNAMENTS

As a kid, I never understood why we didn't have more new ornaments each year. As I grew up, I realized *ornaments are expensive*. Especially for something you use just once a year!

Cinnamon sticks make the perfect holiday DIY material—they're hollow inside, so you can thread string through them; they're sturdy, so they don't break easily; and they're scented, so your whole house will smell sweet!

There are a few ways you can use cinnamon sticks to decorate your house for the holidays. You can create unique ornaments (that cost far less than a store-bought ones!) or simply glue cinnamon sticks to holiday wreaths (or pretty much anything you think needs a little extra cinnamon decoration!).

CINNAMON STICK CHRISTMAS TREE ORNAMENT

4 cinnamon sticks
Red and green buttons or artificial tree bristles (optional)
Cardstock paper in gold or silver
Twine or ribbon

NUTRITION

BEAUTY

HEALTH

HOME

1. Cut three of the cinnamon sticks so you have one large, one medium, and one small.

2. Lay the uncut cinnamon stick vertically on your workspace. Use a hot glue gun to horizontally glue the three sticks you cut onto the vertical stick (put the largest at the bottom and smallest at the top). Try and make sure they're evenly spaced.

3. If you're using buttons, glue them on the horizontal sticks. If you're using artificial tree bristle, cut it so it's the same size as the cinnamon sticks and glue on top of the horizontal sticks.

4. Cut a star shape out of the cardstock. Glue it on top of the tree.

5. Loop a piece of twine and tie the ends together. Glue the knot on the back of the tree.

6. Let dry and hang!

CINNAMON STICK REINDEER ORNAMENT

3 cinnamon sticks
Red bell, button, small pom-pom, or felt (for a nose)
2 googly eyes
Twine

1. Arrange two of the cinnamon sticks together in a V shape (be sure they are touching but not overlapping). Lay the third stick on top horizontally; adjust the sticks until you are satisfied with the shape of the reindeer's face.

2. Use a hot glue gun to glue the three sticks together.

3. Place a dot of glue on the point (bottom) of the V and attach your selected nose.

4. Glue a googly eye on each stick where the horizontal and vertical sticks meet.

5. Loop a piece of twine and tie the ends together. Glue the knot on the back of the reindeer.

6. Let dry and hang!

CINNAMON STICK STAR ORNAMENT

5 cinnamon sticks (evenly sized)

Twine, ribbon, or yarn

1. Create an upside-down V with two of the sticks. Unlike the reindeer, lay one of the sticks on top of the other in the V. Glue them together at the point where the V connects.

2. Glue a third stick horizontally just below the top of the V.

3. With the fourth stick, create a diagonal so the top is touching the left end of the horizontal stick and the bottom is touching the stick making up the right side of the V. Glue on the fourth stick.

4. Lay the fifth stick at the right end of the horizontal stick; bring the other end to the bottom of the stick making up the left side of the V. Glue on the fifth stick.

5. Create a loop of twine around the top of the star; tie off and trim any excess.

6. Let dry and hang!

100. DRINK COASTER

If you want to maintain the smooth surfaces of your kitchen counter, coffee table, nightstand, and dining table, then coffee coasters are a must. When condensation from cool drinks drips onto the table surface, it leaves a mark. And hot drinks can burn the surface they're sitting on, leaving a ring even after you've removed the drink.

Cinnamon coasters are a cheap, easy way to prevent your tables and counters from drink rings. They also add a rustic, woodsy touch to your living room and kitchen.

DRINK COASTER

6 3-inch cinnamon sticks of similar thickness

20 inches of yarn, twine, or strong string

1. Line your cinnamon sticks up evenly. Make sure the smooth side (no crack or open seam) is up.

2. Have someone hold the cinnamon sticks for you (or use a book as weight to keep them down) as you weave the yarn, twine, or string through the sticks.

3. *To weave:* Firmly tie the yarn around the first stick. Bring the yarn **over** the first stick and weave it **under** the second stick, **over** the third stick, **under** the fourth stick, and **over** the fifth stick. Make sure the yarn is tight so the coaster will stay together. Once you get to the last stick, loop around and repeat so each stick has yarn showing on the top side. Tie the yarn together to finish and snip off the remaining yarn.

4. Repeat this on the other end of the coaster. That's it!

101. TISSUE BOX COVER

An easy way to add some personalized decor to your house is to spruce up your tissue boxes; it's a small touch that can add cohesion between the rooms. You can make a tissue box cover with cinnamon sticks—it gives your whole house a festive cinnamon scent and makes the colder months feel a little warmer.

TISSUE BOX COVER

Wooden tissue box

Paint and paintbrush

Cinnamon sticks

Ribbon (optional; I suggest a color that matches the paint you chose)

1. Paint your wooden tissue box with your paint of choice. I suggest autumn-themed colors like burgundy, burnt orange, gold, or forest green. *Note: If you choose gold, it can look pretty to paint the cinnamon sticks gold as well!*
2. Let the paint dry.
3. Begin hot gluing cinnamon sticks on the sides of the box. Depending on the size of the tissue box and the sticks you have, you may want to do two layers.
4. Let the glue dry completely.
5. Tie a ribbon around the box if desired. Put the box over your tissue box and enjoy!

NUTRITION

BEAUTY

HEALTH

HOME

NOTES

INTRODUCTION

1. Alex Delany, "Did You Know That There Are Different Types of Cinnamon?," *Bon Appétit*, September 27, 2018, https://www.bonappetit.com/story/types-of-cinnamon.

2. "Cinnamaldehyde," National Center for Biotechnology Information, PubChem Compound Database, https://pubchem.ncbi.nlm.nih.gov/compound/Cinnamaldehyde.

3. Troy David Osborne, "A Taste of Paradise: Cinnamon," University of Minnesota, https://www.lib.umn.edu/bell/tradeproducts/cinnamon.

4. "Cinnamon," Winchester Hospital, https://www.winchesterhospital.org/health-library/article?id=21672.

CHAPTER 1

1. Pasupuleti Visweswara Rao and Siew Hua Gan, "Cinnamon: A Multifaceted Medicinal Plant," *Evidence-Based Complementary and Alternative Medicine* 2014 (April 2014): 1–12, https://doi.org/10.1155/2014/642942.

2. Anna Davies, "What Is Bulletproof Coffee and Is It Actually Good for You?," Chowhound, January 14, 2020, https://www.chowhound.com/food-news/212150/what-is-bulletproof-coffee-is-it-good-for-you.

3. "The History of Butter," Butter Journal, http://www.butterjournal.com/butter-history.

4. "History Of Food Preservation Timeline: When Did People Start To Preserve Food?," DehydratorLab.com, https://dehydratorlab.com/history-of-food-preservation.

5. Seyed Fazel Nabavi et al., "Antibacterial Effects of Cinnamon: From Farm to Food, Cosmetic and Pharmaceutical Industries," *Nutrients* 7, no. 9 (September 2015): 7729–48, https://doi.org/10.3390/nu7095359.

6. Sean Paajanen, "An Abridged History of Hot Chocolate: Its Changes Over the Years," The Spruce Eats, February 6, 2019, https://www.thespruceeats.com/the-history-of-hot-chocolate-764463.

7. Niamh Michail, "How Mexico's cinnamon-spiked hot chocolate mirrors the country's history," Foodnavigator-latam.com, March 22, 2019, https://www.foodnavigator-latam.com/Article/2019/03/22/How-Mexico-s-cinnamon-spiked-hot-chocolate-mirrors-the-country-s-history.

8. Lindsey Goodwin, "The History of Masala Chai: From Ayurvedic Ambrosia to Americanized Coffeehouse Treat," The Spruce Eats, October 24, 2019, https://www.thespruceeats.com/the-history-of-masala-chai-tea-765836.

9. Lad Vasant, "Ayurveda: A Brief Introduction and Guide," The Ayurvedic Institute, 2006, https://www.ayurveda.com/resources/articles/ayurveda-a-brief-introduction-and-guide.

10. The Ayurveda Experience, "Cinnamon: Everything You Need To Know," The Ayurveda Experience, November 17, 2018, https://www.theayurveda-experience.com/blog/cinnamon-ayurveda.

11. Gaia Herbs, "The Ultimate Guide to Golden Milk, Everything You Need to Know," Gaia Herbs, October 20, 2016, https://www.gaiaherbs.com/blogs/seeds-of-knowledge/the-ultimate-guide-to-golden-milk.

12. VinePair Staff, "A (Brief) History Of The Cocktail," VinePair, https://vinepair.com/spirits-101/history-of-the-cocktail.

13. "History of Spices," McCormick Science Institute, https://www.mccormickscienceinstitute.com/resources/history-of-spices.

14. Y. H Hui et al., eds., *Meat Science and Applications* (New York: Marcel Dekker, 2001).

15. Heather Whipps, "How the Spice Trade Changed the World," LiveScience, May 12, 2008, https://www.livescience.com/7495-spice-trade-changed-world.html.

16. Alam Khan et al., "Cinnamon Improves Glucose and Lipids of People With Type 2 Diabetes," *Diabetes Care* 26, no. 12 (2003): 3215–18, https://doi.org/10.2337/diacare.26.12.3215.

17. Erin Palinski-Wade, "Flour Power: 5 Options That Are Good for Baking and Diabetes," OnTrack Diabetes, November 16, 2016, https://www.ontrackdiabetes.com/blogs/ask-diabetes-nutrition-expert/flour-power-5-options-are-good-baking-diabetes.

18. Mariel Synan, "Cinnamon's Spicy History," History.com, October 4, 2013, https://www.history.com/news/cinnamons-spicy-history.

19. MasterClass, "What Is Cinnamon? How to Cook With Cinnamon Spice," MasterClass, July 2, 2019, https://www.masterclass.com/articles /what-is-cinnamon-how-to-cook-with-cinnamon-spice.

20. Pallavi Kawatra and Rathai Rajagopalan, "Cinnamon: Mystic powers of a minute ingredient," *Pharmacognosy Research* 7, no. 5 (June 2015): 1, https:// doi.org/10.4103/0974-8490.157990.

21. Keith Singletary, "Cinnamon," *Nutrition Today* 54, no. 1 (January 2019): 42–52, https://doi.org/10.1097/nt.0000000000000319.

22. "Cinnamon Intake May Improve Memory," GEN (Genetic Engineering & Biotechnology News), July 22, 2016, https://www.genengnews.com/news /cinnamon-intake-may-improve-memory.

23. Julia Grimaldi, "History of Pickling," Mass Great Outdoors Blog, August 11, 2014, https://blog.mass.gov/greatoutdoors/education/history-of-pickling.

24. Nabavi et al., "Antibacterial Effects of Cinnamon: From Farm to Food, Cosmetic and Pharmaceutical Industries," 7729–48.

25. EricT_CulinaryLore, "What Does Infusion Mean In Cooking?," CulinaryLore, September 23, 2016, https://culinarylore.com /cooking-terms:what-does-infusion-mean-in-cooking.

CHAPTER 2

1. Maria Hernandez-Reif et al., "Breast cancer patients have improved immune and neuroendocrine functions following massage therapy," *Journal of Psychosomatic Research* 57, no. 1 (July 2004): 45–52, https://doi.org/10.1016 /s0022-3999(03)00500-2.

2. "Adults Demonstrate Modified Immune Response After Receiving Massage, Cedars-Sinai Researchers Show," Cedars-Sinai, September 7, 2010, https://www.cedars-sinai.org/newsroom/adults-demonstrate-modified- immune-response-after-receiving-massage-cedars-sinai-researchers-show.

3. Reza Badalzadeh et al., "The Effect of Cinnamon Extract and Long- Term Aerobic Training on Heart Function, Biochemical Alterations and Lipid Profile Following Exhaustive Exercise in Male Rats," *Advanced Pharmaceutical Bulletin* 4, no. 6 (2014): 515–20, https://doi.org/10.5681 /apb.2014.076.

4. Elin Julianti, Kasturi K. Rajah, and Irda Fidrianny, "Antibacterial Activity of Ethanolic Extract of Cinnamon Bark, Honey, and Their Combination Effects against Acne-Causing Bacteria," *Scientia Pharmaceutica* 85, no. 2 (April 2017): 19, https://doi.org/10.3390/scipharm85020019.

5.   Emily Thacker, *The Cinnamon Book* (Hartville, OH: James Direct Inc, 2012).

6.   Gabriella Fabbrocini, Sara Cacciapuoti, and Giuseppe Monfrecola, "A Qualitative Investigation of the Impact of Acne on Health-Related Quality of Life (HRQL): Development of a Conceptual Model," *Dermatology and Therapy* 8, no. 1 (February 2018): 85–99, https://doi.org/10.1007/s13555-018-0224-7.

7.   "Acne: Who Gets and Causes," American Academy of Dermatology, https://www.aad.org/acne-causes.

8.   Emily Gaynor and Kristi Kellogg, "How To Lighten Hair Naturally: 7 Tips for Lighter Hair," Teen Vogue, April 14, 2020, https://www.teenvogue.com/story/how-to-lighten-hair-with-the-sun.

9.   Hallie Levine, "What Actually Happens To Your Hair As You Get Older," Prevention, April 18, 2016, https://www.prevention.com/beauty/a20508421/aging-hair-myths.

10.   Ralph M. Trueb, Hudson Dutra Rezende, and Maria Fernanda Reis Gavazzoni Dias, "A comment on the science of hair aging," *International Journal of Trichology* 10, no. 6 (2018): 245–54, https://doi.org/10.4103/ijt.ijt_56_18.

11.   Laura Indriana, Wimpie Pangkahila, and I. Gusti Made Aman, "Topical application of cinnamon (cinnamomum burmanii) essential oil has the same effectiveness as minoxidil in increasing hair length and diameter size of hair follicles in male white Wistar rats (*rattus norvegicus*)," *Indonesian Journal of Anti-Aging Medicine* 2, no. 1 (January–June 2018): 13–16.

12.   Catherine Devine, "Just the Facts: Cinnamon Oil for Hair Loss," Allure, August 28, 2013, https://www.allure.com/story/does-cinnamon-oil-prevent-hair-loss.

13.   Pallavi Kawatra and Rathai Rajagopalan, "Cinnamon: Mystic powers of a minute ingredient," *Pharmacognosy Research* 7, no. 5 (June 2015): 1, https://doi.org/10.4103/0974-8490.157990.

14.   "Dry Skin," American Osteopathic College of Dermatology (AOCD), https://www.aocd.org/page/DrySkin.

15.   Bruno Burlando and Laura Cornara, "Honey in dermatology and skin care: a review," *Journal of Cosmetic Dermatology* 12, no. 4 (December 2013): 306–13, https://doi.org/10.1111/jocd.12058.

16.   Becky Little, "Arsenic Pills and Lead Foundation: The History of Toxic Makeup," National Geographic, September 22, 2016, https://www.nationalgeographic.com/news/2016/09/ingredients-lipstick-makeup-cosmetics-science-history.

17.   Alanna Martine Kilkeary, "Beauty PI: The Surprising (and Kind of Ugly) History of Foundation," Makeup.com, March 27, 2018, https://www.makeup.com/history-of-makeup-foundation.

18. "Skin Exposures and Effects," Centers for Disease Control and Prevention, July 2, 2013, https://www.cdc.gov/niosh/topics/skin.

19. Health Agenda magazine, "The Importance of Oral Health: Dental hygiene isn't just about teeth, good oral health can also help prevent a number of diseases," HCF, January 2017, https://www.hcf.com.au/health-agenda /health-care/common-conditions/the-importance-of-oral-health.

20. Thomas P. Connelly, "The History of Toothpaste: From 5000 BC to the Present," HuffPost, November 17, 2011, https://www.huffpost.com/entry /mouth-health-the-history-_b_702332.

21. Sebastian G. Ciancio, "Baking soda dentifrices and oral health," *Journal of the American Dental Association* 148, no. 11 (November 2017), https://doi .org/10.1016/j.adaj.2017.09.009.

22. "Minipoo Dry Shampoo," National Museum of American History, https:// americanhistory.si.edu/collections/search/object/nmah_1414219.

23. Alanna Nuñez, "9 Things You Don't Know About Using Dry Shampoo," Reader's Digest, February 10, 2017, https://www.rd.com/beauty /dry-shampoo.

24. Brooke Shunatona, "How to Contour and Highlight for Your Face Shape," Cosmopolitan, March 23, 2020, https://www.cosmopolitan.com /style-beauty/beauty/how-to/a43730/face-shape-contour-map.

25. "What you need to know about alopecia areata," National Alopecia Areata Foundation, https://www.naaf.org/alopecia-areata.

26. Tung-Chou Wen et al., "Effect of *Cinnamomum osmophloeum* Kanehira Leaf Aqueous Extract on Dermal Papilla Cell Proliferation and Hair Growth," *Cell Transplantation* 27, no. 2 (April 2018): 256–63. https://doi .org/10.1177/0963689717741139.

27. *2018 Plastic Surgery Statistics Report*, American Society of Plastic Surgeons, https://www.plasticsurgery.org/documents/News/Statistics/2018/plastic- surgery-statistics-full-report-2018.pdf.

28. Christine Ruggeri, "Cassia Oil Improves Circulation, Arthritis & Depression," Dr. Axe, March 18, 2018. https://draxe.com/essential-oils/cassia-oil.

29. Amy Marturana Winderl, "The Thing Every Woman Gets Wrong About Cellulite," SELF, June 29, 2016, https://www.self.com/story /cellulite-is-way-more-common-than-you-think.

30. Julia Malacoff, "Everything You Ever Wanted to Know About Cellulite," Shape, https://www.shape.com/weight-loss/tips-plans/what-cellulite.

31. "Cellulite Treatments: What Really Works?," American Academy of Dermatology, https://www.aad.org/public/cosmetic/fat-removal /cellulite-treatments-what-really-works.

32. Ashley Houk, "The Benefits of Dry Brushing," Mother Earth Living, https://www.motherearthliving.com/real-beauty/benefits-of-dry-brushing -zb0z1611zhou.

33. Jessica Chia, "Can Caffeine Really Help Reduce Cellulite?," Women's Health, March 24, 2016, https://www.womenshealthmag.com/beauty/a19938541 /treating-cellulite-with-caffeine/.

34. "Acne: Who Gets and Causes," American Academy of Dermatology.

35. Tash, "The Complete List of Comedogenic Oils," Holistic Health Herbalist, https://www.holistichealthherbalist.com/complete-list-of-comedogenic -oils.

36. "Uses and benefits of Epsom salt," Epsom Salt Council, https://www.epsom-saltcouncil.org/uses-benefits.

37. "History of Soap and Soap Interesting Facts," Soap History, http://www.soa-phistory.net.

38. Jenna Rosenstein, "Are Bath Bombs Actually Good for Your Skin?," Allure, September 10, 2017, https://www.allure.com/story /do-bath-bombs-really-work.

39. Vivian Manning-Schaffel, "How to heal dry, cracked heels, according to dermatologists," BETTER by TODAY, November 14, 2019, https://www.nbcnews.com/better/lifestyle/how-care-dry-cracked-heels-according -dermatologists-ncna1080001.

40. Karim Orange, "Anti-Aging Part One: The Importance of Collagen," HuffPost, November 28, 2016, https://www.huffpost.com/entry/anti -aging-part-1-the-importance-of-collagen_b_583cd543e4b04e28cf5b8ac3>.

41. Naoko Takasao et al., "Cinnamon Extract Promotes Type I Collagen Biosynthesis via Activation of IGF-I Signaling in Human Dermal Fibroblasts," *Journal of Agricultural and Food Chemistry* 60, no. 5 (January 2012): 1193–200, https://doi.org/10.1021/jf2043357.

42. Takasao, "Cinnamon Extract Promotes Type I Collagen Biosynthesis via Activation of IGF-I Signaling in Human Dermal Fibroblasts," 1193–200.

43. "Harmful effects of ultraviolet radiation. Council on Scientific Affairs," *The Journal of the American Medical Association* 262, no. 3 (July 1989): 380–84, PMID: 2661872; "Tanning & Your Skin," Skin Cancer Foundation, June 2019, https://www.skincancer.org/risk-factors/tanning.

CHAPTER 3

1. A.H. Atta and A. Alkofahi, "Anti-nociceptive and anti-inflamma-tory effects of some Jordanian medicinal plant extracts," *Journal of Ethnopharmacology* 60, no. 2 (March 1998): 117–24, https://doi.org/10.1016/ s0378-8741(97)00137-2.

2. Martina Morokutti-Kurz, Christine Graf, and Eva Prieschl-Grassauer, "Amylmetacresol/2,4-dichlorobenzyl alcohol, hexylresorcinol, or carrageenan lozenges as active treatments for sore throat," *International Journal of General Medicine* 2017, no. 10 (February 2017): 53–60, https://doi.org/10.2147/ijgm.s120665.

3. Manisha Deb Mandal and Shyamapada Mandal, "Honey: its medicinal property and antibacterial activity," *Asian Pacific Journal of Tropical Biomedicine* 1, no. 2 (April 2011): 154–60, https://doi.org/10.1016/s2221-1691(11)60016-6.

4. Seyed Fazel Nabavi et al., "Antibacterial Effects of Cinnamon: From Farm to Food, Cosmetic and Pharmaceutical Industries," *Nutrients* 7, no. 9 (September 2015): 7729–48, https://doi.org/10.3390/nu7095359.

5. D. A. Vattem et al., "Dietary supplementation with two Lamiaceae herbs-(oregano and sage) modulates innate immunity parameters in *Lumbricus terrestris*," *Pharmacognosy Research* 5, no. 1 (2013): 1–9, https://doi.org/10.4103/0974-8490.105636.

6. "Dextromethorphan (DXM)," CESAR, http://www.cesar.umd.edu/cesar/drugs/dxm.asp.

7. Saeed Samarghandian, Tahereh Farkhondeh, and Fariborz Samini, "Honey and Health: A Review of Recent Clinical Research," *Pharmacognosy Research* 9, no. 2 (April–June 2017): 121–27, https://doi.org/10.4103/0974-8490.204647.

8. "Mouthwash (Mouthrinse)," American Dental Association, August 29, 2019, https://www.ada.org/en/member-center/oral-health-topics/mouthrinse.

9. Sebastian G. Ciancio, "Baking soda dentifrices and oral health," *Journal of the American Dental Association* 148, no. 11 (November 2017), https://doi.org/10.1016/j.adaj.2017.09.009.

10. Vagish Kumar L. Shanbhag, "Oil pulling for maintaining oral hygiene—A review," *Journal of Traditional and Complementary Medicine* 7, no. 1 (January 2017): 106–09, https://doi.org/10.1016/j.jtcme.2016.05.004.

11. "Athlete's foot: Overview," InformedHealth.org [Internet], June 14, 2018, https://www.ncbi.nlm.nih.gov/books/NBK279549.

12. Jolene Feldman and Immanuel Barshi, *The Effects of Blood Glucose Levels on Cognitive Performance: A Review of the Literature*, NASA (National Aeronautics and Space Administration), 2007.

13. "Cinnamon may be fragrant medicine for the brain," U.S. Department of Veterans Affairs, July 21, 2016, https://www.research.va.gov/currents/0716-6.cfm.

14. Mandal and Mandal, "Honey: its medicinal property and antibacterial activity," 154–60.

15. "Why Do We Eat Chicken Noodle Soup When We Are Sick?," UPMC HealthBeat, February 15, 2014, https://share.upmc.com/2014/02/chicken-noodle-soup-when-sick.

16. Josh Axe, "5 Signs You're Suffering From Candida Overgrowth—and What You Can Do About It," U.S. News & World Report, https://health.usnews .com/health-news/blogs/eat-run/articles/2015-12-23/5-signs-youre-suffer-ing-from-candida-overgrowth-and-what-you-can-do-about-it.

17. "Vaginal candidiasis," Centers for Disease Control and Prevention, December 17, 2019, https://www.cdc.gov/fungal/diseases/candidiasis/genital.

18. "Which Countries Have the Highest and Lowest Cancer Rates? [Updated 2019]," Dana-Farber Cancer Institute, September 30, 2019, https://blog .dana-farber.org/insight/2019/09/which-countries-have-the-highest-and-lowest-cancer-rates.

19. Ho-Keun Kwon et al., "Cinnamon extract suppresses tumor progression by modulating angiogenesis and the effector function of CD8$^+$ T cells," *Cancer Letters* 278, no. 2 (June 2009): 174–82, https://doi.org/10.1016/j .canlet.2009.01.015.

20. Shahla Kakoei et al., "Prevalence of Toothache and Associated Factors: A Population-Based Study in Southeast Iran," *Iranian Endodontic Journal* 8, no. 3 (Summer 2013): 123–28, PMID: 23922574.

21. "Toothache," Cleveland Clinic, March 23, 2020, https://my.clevelandclinic .org/health/diseases/10957-toothache.

22. D. L. Nurmalasari, M. Damiyanti, and Y. K. Eriwati, "Effect of cinnamon extract solution on human tooth enamel surface roughness," *Journal of Physics: Conference Series* 1073, no. 3 (2018): 032022, https://doi .org/10.1088/1742-6596/1073/3/032022.

23. Jian Zhen Ou et al., "Potential of *in vivo* real-time gastric gas profiling: a pilot evaluation of heat-stress and modulating dietary cinnamon effect in an animal model," *Scientific Reports* 6, no. 33387 (September 2016), https:// www.nature.com/articles/srep33387.

24. Pallavi Kawatra and Rathai Rajagopalan, "Cinnamon: Mystic powers of a minute ingredient," *Pharmacognosy Research* 7, no. 5 (June 2015): 1, https:// doi.org/10.4103/0974-8490.157990; Mariel Synan, "Cinnamon's Spicy History," History.com, October 4, 2013, https://www.history.com/news /cinnamons-spicy-history.

25. Esther Muchene, "6 natural home remedies for passing gas," Eve, https:// www.standardmedia.co.ke/evewoman/article/2001265490/6-natural-home -remedies-for-passing-gas.

26. Alessandro Villa, "Bad breath: What causes it and what to do about it," Harvard Health, January 21, 2019, https://www.health.harvard.edu/blog /bad-breath-what-causes-it-and-what-to-do-about-it-2019012115803.

27. "Definition and Symptoms of Chronic Kidney Disease," DaVita, https://inter-national.davita.com/pl/en/patient-resources/kidney-disease-education /symptoms-and-diagnoses/10067.

28. "Researchers Improve Wound Healing with Cinnamon Treatment," Advanced Tissue, June 23, 2016, https://advancedtissue.com/2016/06/researchers-improve-wound-healing-with-cinnamon-treatment.

29. "Peppermint oil and cinnamon could help treat and heal chronic wounds," American Chemical Society, July 8, 2015, https://www.acs.org/content/acs/en/pressroom/presspacs/2015/acs-presspac-july-8-2015/peppermint-oil-and-cinnamon-could-help-treat-and-heal-chronic-wounds.html.

30. S. Siddiqua et al., "Antibacterial activity of cinnamaldehyde and clove oil: effect on selected foodborne pathogens in model food systems and watermelon juice," Journal of Food Science and Technology 52, no. 9 (November 2014): 5834–41, https://doi.org/10.1007/s13197-014-1642-x.

31. Peter Molan and Tanya Rhodes, "Honey: A Biologic Wound Dressing," Wounds 27, no. 6 (June 2015): 141–51, https://www.woundsresearch.com/article/honey-biologic-wound-dressing; "Researchers Improve Wound Healing with Cinnamon Treatment."

32. Jessica Brown, "What we do and don't know about gut health," BBC Future, January 22, 2019, https://www.bbc.com/future/article/20190121-what-we-do-and-dont-know-about-gut-health.

33. Jo Lewin, "The health benefits of cinnamon," BBC Good Food, September 13, 2019, https://www.bbcgoodfood.com/howto/guide/health-benefits-cinnamon.

34. "What is Eczema?," National Eczema Association, https://nationaleczema.org/eczema.

35. "Eczema Causes and Triggers," National Eczema Association, https://nationaleczema.org/eczema/causes-and-triggers-of-eczema.

36. Rajani Katta and Megan Schlichte, "Diet and Dermatitis: Food Triggers," Journal of Clinical and Aesthetic Dermatology 7, no. 3 (March 2014): 30–36, PMID: 24688624.

37. "Heart Disease Facts," Centers for Disease Control and Prevention, June 22, 2020, https://www.cdc.gov/heartdisease/facts.htm.

38. "HDL (Good), LDL (Bad) Cholesterol and Triglycerides," American Heart Association, April 30, 2017, https://www.heart.org/en/health-topics/cholesterol/hdl-good-ldl-bad-cholesterol-and-triglycerides; "Could Too Much 'Good' HDL Cholesterol Be Bad for Your Heart?," South Lake Women's Healthcare, August 27, 2018, https://southlakewomens.com/blog/could-too-much-good-hdl-cholesterol-be-bad-for-your-heart.

39. "11 foods that lower cholesterol," Harvard Health, October 2009, https://www.health.harvard.edu/heart-health/11-foods-that-lower-cholesterol.

40. "Why You Should Have a Daily Dose of Cinnamon," Good Housekeeping, January 16, 2014, https://www.goodhousekeeping.com/health/diet-nutrition/a19907/cinnamon-benefits.

41. "Statistics About Diabetes," American Diabetes Association, https://www
.diabetes.org/resources/statistics/statistics-about-diabetes.

42. Alam Khan et al., "Cinnamon Improves Glucose and Lipids of People With
Type 2 Diabetes," *Diabetes Care* 26, no. 12 (2003): 3215–18, https://doi
.org/10.2337/diacare.26.12.3215.

43. Robert W. Allen et al., "Cinnamon Use in Type 2 Diabetes: An Updated
Systematic Review and Meta-Analysis," *Annals of Family Medicine* 11, no. 5
(September 2013): 452–59, https://doi.org/10.1370/afm.1517.

44. Shahla Fadaei and Masoomeh Asle-Rousta, "Anxiolytic and antidepressant
effects of cinnamon (Cinnamomum verum) extract in rats receiving lead
acetate," *Scientific Journal of Kurdistan University of Medical Sciences* 22, no.
6 (October 2018): 31–39, https://doi.org/10.22102/22.6.31.

45. Isa Kay, "Is Your Mood Disorder a Symptom of Unstable Blood Sugar?,"
Univeristy of Michigan, School of Public Health, October 21, 2019, https://
sph.umich.edu/pursuit/2019posts/mood-blood-sugar-kujawski.html.

46. Therese Borchard, "10 Fall Foods to Boost Your Mood," EverydayHealth,
October   6,   2016,   https://www.everydayhealth.com/columns/therese
-borchard-sanity-break/10-fall-foods-to-boost-your-mood.

47. Uma Naidoo, "Gut feelings: How food affects your mood," Harvard Health,
December 7, 2018, https://www.health.harvard.edu/blog/gut-feelings-how
-food-affects-your-mood-2018120715548.

48. Sumanta Kumar Goswami et al., "Efficacy of Cinnamomum cassia Blume. in
age induced sexual dysfunction of rats," *Journal of Young Pharmacists* 5, no.
4 (2013): 148–53, https://doi.org/10.1016/j.jyp.2013.11.001.

49. "What Is Arthritis?," Arthritis Foundation, https://www.arthritis.org
/health-wellness/about-arthritis/understanding-arthritis/what-is-arthritis.

50. Kentaro Tsuji-Naito, "Aldehydic components of Cinnamon bark extract
suppresses RANKL-induced osteoclastogenesis through NFATc1 down-
regulation," *Bioorganic & Medicinal Chemistry* 16, no. 20 (October 2008):
9176–183, https://doi.org/10.1016/j.bmc.2008.09.036.

51. Pasupuleti Visweswara Rao and Siew Hua Gan, "Cinnamon: A Multifaceted
Medicinal Plant," *Evidence-Based Complementary and Alternative Medicine*
2014 (April 2014): 1–12, https://doi.org/10.1155/2014/642942.

52. "Best Spices for Arthritis," Arthritis Foundation, https://www.arthritis.
org/health-wellness/healthy-living/nutrition/healthy-eating/best-spices
-for-arthritis.

53. Rebecca C. Brown, Alan H. Lockwood, and Babasaheb R. Sonawane,
"Neurodegenerative Diseases: An Overview of Environmental Risk Factors,"
Environmental Health Perspectives 113, no. 9 (September 2005): 1250–256,
https://doi.org/10.1289/ehp.7567.

54. Brown, Lockwood, and Sonawane, "Neurodegenerative Diseases: An Overview of Environmental Risk Factors," 1250–56; Sabrian Giacoppo et al., "Heavy Metals and Neurodegenerative Diseases: An Observational Study," *Biological Trace Element Research* 161 (August 2014): 151–60, https://doi.org/10.1007/s12011-014-0094-5.

55. "What Happens to the Brain in Alzheimer's Disease?," National Institute on Aging, May 16, 2017, https://www.nia.nih.gov/health/what-happens-brain-alzheimers-disease.

56. Dylan W. Peterson et al., "Cinnamon Extract Inhibits Tau Aggregation Associated with Alzheimer's Disease In Vitro," *Journal of Alzheimer's Disease* 17, no. 3 (July 2009): 585–97, https://doi.org/10.3233/jad-2009-1083.

57. "Causes: Parkinson's disease," NHS, April 30, 2019, https://www.nhs.uk/conditions/parkinsons-disease/causes/.

58. Rush University Medical Center, "Cinnamon may be used to halt progression of Parkinson's disease, study suggests," ScienceDaily, July 9, 2014, https://www.sciencedaily.com/releases/2014/07/140709095257.htm.

59. "What is Osteoporosis and What Causes It?," National Osteoporosis Foundation, https://www.nof.org/patients/what-is-osteoporosis.

60. "Cinnamon Inhibits Osteoclasts In Vitro," Osteoporosis-Studies, September 5, 2013, http://osteoporosis-studies.com/category/supplements/cinnamon.

61. Steven L. Teitelbaum, "Osteoclasts: What Do They Do and How Do They Do It?" *American Journal of Pathology* 170, no. 2 (February 2007): 427–35, https://doi.org/10.2353/ajpath.2007.060834.

62. Prashant Singh, Sonia S. Yoon, and Braden Kuo, "Nausea: a review of pathophysiology and therapeutics," *Therapeutic Advances in Gastroenterology* 9, no. 1 (November 2015): 98–112, https://doi.org/10.1177/1756283x15618131.

63. Anu Saini, "Evidence-Based Home remedies for Nausea," Ayur Times, November 14, 2016, https://www.ayurtimes.com/nausea-home-remedies.

64. Karen Mustian et al., "Treatment of Nausea and Vomiting During Chemotherapy," *US Oncology & Hematology*, 7, no. 2 (January 2011): 91–97, https://doi.org/10.17925/ohr.2011.07.2.91.

65. Molouk Jaafarpour et al., "The Effect of Cinnamon on Menstrual Bleeding and Systemic Symptoms With Primary Dysmenorrhea," *Iranian Red Crescent Medical Journal* 17, no. 4 (April 2015): e59647, https://doi.org/10.5812/ircmj.17(4)2015.27032.

66. Amber Scriven, "7 Herbal Remedies That Can Help Relieve A Stiff Neck, According To An Herbalist & Acupuncturist," Mindbodygreen, March 30, 2020, https://www.mindbodygreen.com/0-5614/7-Natural-Tricks-to-Heal-a-Stiff-Neck.html.

67. A. Narayanan et al., "Oral supplementation of *trans*-cinnamaldehyde reduces uropathogenic *Escherichia coli* colonization in a mouse model," *Letters in Applied Microbiology* 64, no. 3 (January 2017): 192–97, https://doi .org/10.1111/lam.12713.

68. "What is a Urinary Tract Infection (UTI) in Adults?," Urology Care Foundation, April 2019, https://www.urologyhealth.org/urologic-conditions /urinary-tract-infections-in-adults.

69. Narayanan, "Oral supplementation of *trans*-cinnamaldehyde reduces uropathogenic *Escherichia coli* colonization in a mouse model," 192–97.

70. "What is a Urinary Tract Infection (UTI) in Adults?," Urology Care Foundation.

71. Kathleen M. Zelman, "The Grapefruit Diet," https://www.medicinenet.com /the_grapefruit_diet/views.htm.

72. Ken Fujioka et al., "The Effects of Grapefruit on Weight and Insulin Resistance: Relationship to the Metabolic Syndrome," *Journal of Medicinal Food* 9, no. 1 (March 2006): 49–54, https://doi.org/10.1089/jmf.2006.9.49.

73. Brian Wilmovsky, *Dream Health: How to Live a Balanced and Healthy Life in an Unbalanced World* (Lake Mary, FL: Siloam, 2006).

74. Caroline J. Cederquist, "Insulin Resistance: The Real Reason Why You Aren't Losing Weight," HuffPost, February 5, 2015, https://www.huffpost.com /entry/metabolism-dysfunction-th_b_6430370.

75. Juan Jiang et al., "Cinnamaldehyde induces fat cell-autonomous thermogenesis and metabolic reprogramming," *Metabolism* 77 (August 2017): 58–64, https://doi.org/10.1016/j.metabol.2017.08.006.

76. David A. Wiss, Nicole Avena, and Pedro Rada, "Sugar Addiction: From Evolution to Revolution," *Frontiers in Psychiatry* 9 (November 2018), https:// doi.org/10.3389/fpsyt.2018.00545.

77. Richard A. Anderson, "Chromium and polyphenols from cinnamon improve insulin sensitivity: Plenary Lecture," *Proceedings of the Nutrition Society* 67, no. 1 (February 2008): 48–53, https://doi.org/10.1017/s0029665108006010.

78. Joan Kent, "How to Handle Sugar Cravings and Recover from Sugar Addiction," TheDiabetesCouncil.com, June 2, 2020, https://www.thediabetescouncil.com/handle-sugar-cravings-recover-sugar-addiction.

79. "Cholesterol," Centers for Disease Control and Prevention, February 21, 2020, https://www.cdc.gov/cholesterol/index.htm.

80. "Your Blood Lipids," University of California, San Francisco, https://dtc. ucsf.edu/living-with-diabetes/diet-and-nutrition/understanding-fats-oils /your-blood-lipids/.

81. Khan, "Cinnamon Improves Glucose and Lipids of People With Type 2 Diabetes," 3215–218.

82. Jennifer Moll, "Can Taking Cinnamon Lower Your Cholesterol?," Verywell Health, January 25, 2020, https://www.verywellhealth.com/can-cinnamon -lower-cholesterol-698109.

83. "FDA advises patients on use of non-steroidal anti-inflammatory drugs (NSAIDs) for COVID-19," U.S. Food & Drug Administration, March 19, 2020, https://www.fda.gov/drugs/drug-safety-and-availability/fda-advises -patients-use-non-steroidal-anti-inflammatory-drugs-nsaids-covid-19.

84. Pat Anson, "Is Cinnamon a Safer Pain Reliever?," Pain News Network, July 13, 2015, https://www.painnewsnetwork.org/stories/2015/7/13/is-cinnamon -a-safer-pain-reliever.

85. Pallavi Latthe, Rita Champaneria, and Khalid Khan, "Dysmenorrhea," *American Family Physician* 85, no. 4 (February 2012): 386–87, https://www .aafp.org/afp/2012/0215/p386.html.

86. Jaafarpour et al., "Effect of Cinnamon on Menstrual Bleeding and Systemic Symptoms With Primary Dysmenorrhea," e59647.

87. Molouk Jaafarpour et al., "Comparative Effect of Cinnamon and Ibuprofen for Treatment of Primary Dysmenorrhea: A Randomized Double-Blind Clinical Trial," *Journal of Clinical and Diagnostic Research* 9, no. 4 (April 2015): QC04–07, https://doi.org/10.7860/jcdr/2015/12084.5783.

88. "PCOS (Polycystic Ovary Syndrome) and Diabetes," Centers for Disease Control and Prevention, March 24, 2020, https://www.cdc.gov/diabetes /basics/pcos.html.

89. Lei Dou et al., "The effect of cinnamon on polycystic ovary syndrome in a mouse model," *Reproductive Biology and Endocrinology* 16, no. 1 (October 2018), https://doi.org/10.1186/s12958-018-0418-y.

90. "Overview of the Immune System," National Institute of Allergy and Infectious Diseases, December 30, 2013, https://www.niaid.nih.gov /research/immune-system-overview.

91. Franziska Roth-Walter et al., "Immune Suppressive Effect of Cinnamaldehyde Due to Inhibition of Proliferation and Induction of Apoptosis in Immune Cells: Implications in Cancer," *PLOS ONE* 9, no. 10 (October 2014), https:// doi.org/10.1371/journal.pone.0108402.

92. F. E. G. Cox, "History of Human Parasitology," *Clinical Microbiology Reviews* 15, no. 4 (October 2002): 595–612, https://doi.org/10.1128/cmr.15 .4.595-612.2002.

93. Todd Watts and Jay Davidson, "12 Best Essential Oils For Parasite Cleansing," Detox Learning Center, January 16, 2019, https://microbeformulas.com /blogs/microbe-formulas/12-best-essential-oils-for-parasite-cleansing.

94. Evan C. Palmer-Young et al., "Effects of the floral phytochemical eugenol on parasite evolution and bumble bee infection and preference," *Scientific Reports* 8, 2074 (February 2018), https://www.nature.com/articles /s41598-018-20369-2?proof=t.

CHAPTER 4

1. Kaitlin Benedict et al., "Estimation of Direct Healthcare Costs of Fungal Diseases in the United States," *Clinical Infectious Diseases* 68, no. 11 (June 2019): 1791–97, https://doi.org/10.1093/cid/ciy776.

2. Mi-Young Yoon, Byeongjin Cha, and Jin-Cheol Kim, "Recent Trends in Studies on Botanical Fungicides in Agriculture," *Plant Pathology Journal* 29, no. 1 (March 2013): 1–9, https://doi.org/10.5423/ppj.rw.05.2012.0072.

3. "Using Cinnamon in the Garden," Growing Organic, https://growingorganic.com/diy-guide/using-cinnamon-in-the-garden.

4. Marie Iannotti, "Damping off Disease of Seedlings," The Spruce, June 10, 2020, https://www.thespruce.com/damping-off-disease-of-seedlings-1402519.

5. Jolanta Kowalska et al., "Cinnamon powder: an in vitro and in vivo evaluation of antifungal and plant growth promoting activity," *European Journal of Plant Pathology* 156, no. 1 (November 2019): 237–43, https://doi .org/10.1007/s10658-019-01882-0.

6. Jon VanZile, "How to Use Powdered Rooting Hormone: Propagating Your Plants From Cuttings," The Spruce, August 7, 2020, https://www.thespruce. com/how-to-use-rooting-hormone-1902934.

7. Society for Neuroscience, "Controlling fire ants with natural compounds," ScienceDaily, February 5, 2018, https://www.sciencedaily.com /releases/2018/02/180205141122.htm.

8. "Mosquito-Borne Diseases," Centers for Disease Control and Prevention, March 21, 2016, https://www.cdc.gov/niosh/topics/outdoor/mosquito -borne/default.html.

9. Adelina Thomas et al., "Evaluation of active ingredients and larvicidal activity of clove and cinnamon essential oils against *Anopheles gambiae* (*sensu lato*)," *Parasites & Vectors* 10, no. 1 (September 2017), https://doi .org/10.1186/s13071-017-2355-6.

10. "All-Natural Room Spray," Martha Stewart, https://www.marthastewart .com/1526211/natural-room-spray-with-essential-oils.

11. "History," National Candle Association, https://candles.org/history.

12. Christine Blume, Corrado Garbazza, and Manuel Spitschan, "Effects of light on human circadian rhythms, sleep and mood," *Somnologie* 23, no. 3 (August 2019): 147–56, https://doi.org/10.1007/s11818-019-00215-x.

13. Lindsay Holmes, "11 Scents That Can Do Wonders For Your Well-Being," HuffPost, April 26, 2014, https://www.huffpost.com/entry/scents-and -wellbeing_n_5193609.

14. BH&G Editors, "How to Clean Almost Every Surface of Your Home With Vinegar," Better Homes & Gardens, March 10, 2020, https://www.bhg.com /homekeeping/house-cleaning/tips/cleaning-with-vinegar.

15. Yunbin Zhang et al., "Antibacterial activity and mechanism of cinnamon essential oil against *Escherichia coli* and *Staphylococcus aureus*," *Food Control* 59 (January 2016): 282–89, https://www.sciencedirect.com/science/article /abs/pii/S0956713515300219.

16. "How to Make Your Car Smell Great Again," Carwise, September 28, 2018, https://www.carwise.com/blog/2018/06/12/how-to-make-your-car-smell -great-again.

17. Ayn-Monique Klahre, "How To Deodorize Your Carpet Naturally with Baking Soda," Kitchn, December 12, 2017, https://www.thekitchn.com /how-to-deodorize-your-carpet-naturally-with-baking-soda-252554.

18. Kathy Keville, "Aromatherapy: Cinnamon," HowStuffWorks, https://health. howstuffworks.com/wellness/natural-medicine/aromatherapy/aromathera- py-cinnamon.htm.

19. "Why Do Mosquitoes Bite Me So Much?," Terminix, https://www.terminix .com/blog/education/why-mosquitoes-bite-me-so-much.

20. Susan Brink, "A Guide To Mosquito Repellents, From DEET To . . . Gin And Tonic?," NPR, June 30, 2018, https://www.npr.org/sections/goatsand- soda/2018/06/30/623865454/a-guide-to-mosquito-repellents-from -deet-to-gin-and-tonic.

21. American Chemical Society, "Cinnamon Oil Kills Mosquitoes," ScienceDaily, July 16, 2004, https://www.sciencedaily.com/releases/2004/07 /040716081706.htm.

22. Michael F. Potter, "Clothes Moths," Entomology at the University of Kentucky, https://entomology.ca.uky.edu/ef609.

23. "Health Effects of Mothballs," National Pesticide Information Center, February 9, 2017, http://npic.orst.edu/ingred/ptype/mothball/health.html.

24. Pest Republic, "How to Get Rid of Moths Naturally," Pest Republic, May 4, 2019, https://pestrepublic.com/how-to-get-rid-of-moths-naturally.

25. Markham Heid, "The Creepy Truth About Humidifiers," Time, March 01, 2017, https://time.com/4685972/humidifier-disinfectants-bacteria-water.

26. Anne Steinemann, "Ten questions concerning air fresheners and indoor built environments," *Building and Environment* 111 (January 2017): 279–84, https://www.sciencedirect.com/science/article/pii/S0360132316304334.

27. F. Gayle Gregory, "Potpourri," Grower Direct, https://www.growerdirect.com/potpourri.

28. Seyed Fazel Nabavi et al., "Antibacterial Effects of Cinnamon: From Farm to Food, Cosmetic and Pharmaceutical Industries," *Nutrients* 7, no. 9 (September 2015): 7729–48, https://doi.org/10.3390/nu7095359.

29. "The History Of The Broom," Spring Wolf, http://www.paganspath.com/magik/broom.htm.

30. "Fed Up With Smelly Shoes? 5 Steps To Fight The Funk Once And For All," Road Runner Sports, https://www.roadrunnersports.com/blog/smelly-shoes.

31. Nabavi, "Antibacterial Effects of Cinnamon: From Farm to Food, Cosmetic and Pharmaceutical Industries," 7729–48.

ABOUT THE AUTHOR

NANCY CHEN is a wellness blogger, content creator, and fitness instructor with a family background in herbal medicine. She's known for creating easy-to-follow recipes and giving effective health and lifestyle guidance on her blog, *Nourish by Nancy*; she currently resides in Santa Monica, California.

AB♦UT FAMILIUS

VISIT OUR WEBSITE: WWW.FAMILIUS.COM
JOIN ♦UR FAMILY

There are lots of ways to connect with us! Subscribe to our newsletters at www.familius.com to receive uplifting daily inspiration, essays from our Pater Familius, a free ebook every month, and the first word on special discounts and Familius news.

GET BULK DISCOUNTS

If you feel a few friends and family might benefit from what you've read, let us know and we'll be happy to provide you with quantity discounts. Simply email us at orders@familius.com.

CONNECT

Facebook: www.facebook.com/paterfamilius
Twitter: @familiustalk, @paterfamilius1
Pinterest: www.pinterest.com/familius
Instagram: @familiustalk

FAMILIUS

> THE M♦ST IMPORTANT W♦RK Y♦U
> EVER DO WILL BE WITHIN THE
> WALLS OF Y♦UR ♦WN HOME.